Contents

Contributing authors iv
Acknowledgements v
Foreword vi
Clinical audit in the NHS: a statement from the National Institute for Clinical Excellence viii

Introduction: using the method, creating the environment 1
Stage One: preparing for audit 9
Stage Two: selecting criteria 21
Stage Three: measuring level of performance 33
Stage Four: making improvements 47
Stage Five: sustaining improvement 59

Appendix I: glossary 69
Appendix II: online resources for clinical audit 73
Appendix III: national audit projects sponsored by the National Institute for Clinical Excellence 93
Appendix IV: further reading 97
Appendix V: key points and key notes 101
Appendix VI: checklists 105
Appendix VII: approach to examining clinical audit during a clinical governance review used by the Commission for Health Improvement 115
Appendix VIII: recommendations from the *Report of the Public Inquiry into Children's Heart Surgery at the Bristol Royal Infirmary 1984–1995* (2001) and the Government's response (2002) 119
Appendix IX: lessons learnt from the National Sentinel Audit Programme 125
Appendix X: list of desirable characteristics of review criteria 131
Appendix XI: review of the evidence 133

Index 191

Contributing authors

Royal College of Nursing
20 Cavendish Square
London, W1G 0RN

Ross Scrivener, Information Manager, *Quality Improvement Programme*

RCN Institute
Radcliffe Infirmary
Oxford, OX2 6HE

Clare Morrell, Senior Research and Development Fellow, *Quality Improvement Programme*

Clinical Governance Research and Development Unit
Department of General Practice and Primary Health Care
University of Leicester
Leicester General Hospital
Gwendolen Road
Leicester, LE5 4PW

Richard Baker, Professor and Director
Sarah Redsell, Senior Lecturer
Elizabeth Shaw, Research Associate
Keith Stevenson, Lecturer

National Institute for Clinical Excellence
11 Strand
London, WC2N 5HR

David Pink, Audit Programme Director
Nicki Bromwich, Audit Development Manager

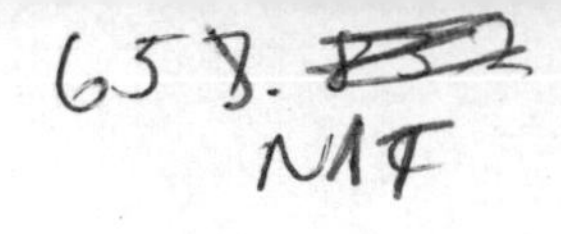

Principles for Best Practice in Clinical Audit

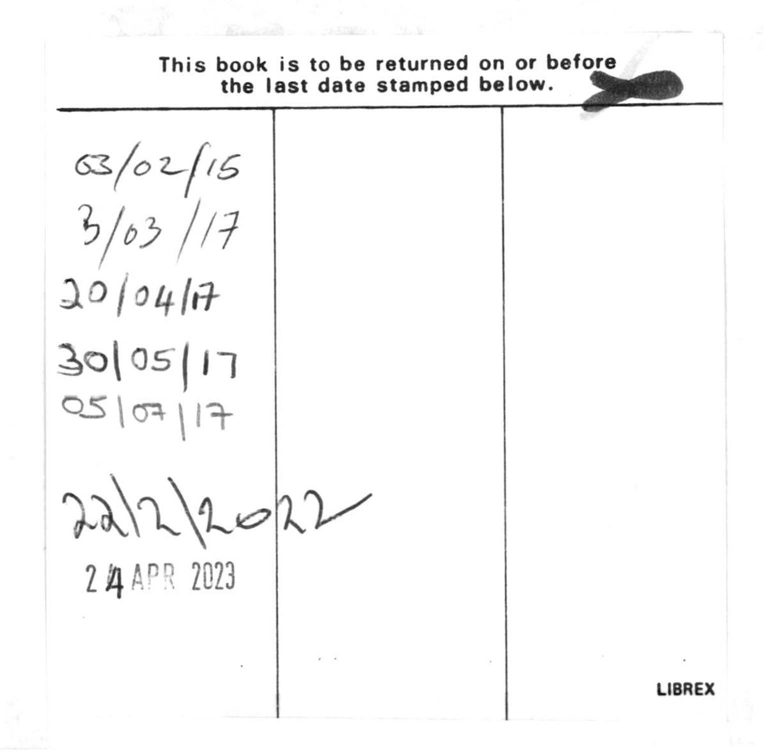

Radcliffe Medical Press

Radcliffe Medical Press Ltd
18 Marcham Road
Abingdon
Oxon OX14 1AA
United Kingdom

www.radcliffe-oxford.com
The Radcliffe Medical Press electronic catalogue and online ordering facility.
Direct sales to anywhere in the world.

Reprinted 2002

British Library Cataloguing in Publication Data

A catalogue record for this book is available from the British Library.

ISBN 1 85775 976 1

Typeset by Aarontype Ltd, Easton, Bristol
Printed and bound by TJ International Ltd, Padstow, Cornwall

Acknowledgements

The preparation of this book was funded by the National Institute for Clinical Excellence. We would like to thank Steve Barrett and Paul Sinfield formerly of CGRDU, Leicester, for assistance in the early stages of the literature review, and Laura Price, for her work in editing the text of the book. Finally, we thank all those – too numerous to mention by name – who reviewed the book during its development.

Foreword

The time has come for everyone in the NHS to take clinical audit very seriously. Anything less would miss the opportunity we now have to re-establish the confidence and trust upon which the NHS is founded.

Public and professional belief in the essential quality of clinical care has been hit hard in recent years, not least by a number of highly public failures. We can no longer think about effectiveness of care as an isolated professional matter. Clinical governance is the organisational approach for quality that integrates the perspectives of staff, patients and their carers, and those charged with managing our health service. But real commitment is needed from everyone involved if governance is to fulfil its promise.

Concerns about the quality of NHS care have attracted national publicity, public inquiries and a focus on failure. While we must do everything we can to put in place systems to avoid such failings in future, these isolated cases should not dominate our thinking about quality of care. It is just as important that clinical governance should support a process of continuous quality improvement throughout the NHS.

Clinical audit is at the heart of clinical governance.

- It provides the mechanisms for reviewing the quality of everyday care provided to patients with common conditions like asthma or diabetes.
- It builds on a long history of doctors, nurses and other healthcare professionals reviewing case notes and seeking ways to serve their patients better.
- It addresses quality issues systematically and explicitly, providing reliable information.
- It can confirm the quality of clinical services and highlight the need for improvement.

This book provides clear statements of principle about clinical audit in the NHS. The authors have reviewed the literature concerned with the development of audit over recent years, and are able to speak about clinical audit with considerable personal authority.

Too often in the past local and national clinical audits have failed to bring about change. The *Report of the Public Inquiry into Children's Heart Surgery at the Bristol Royal Infirmary 1984–1995* (2001) provides salutary reading for anyone in the NHS who is still inclined to dismiss the importance of clinical audit. But audit cannot be expected to bear fruit unless it takes place within a supportive organisation committed to a mature approach to clinical quality – clinical governance.

Clinical audit does not provide a straightforward or guaranteed solution for each problem. Local audit programmes in primary and secondary care will need to use the principles set out in this book to devise and agree local programmes tailored to address local issues. Nevertheless, we hope you will find that the distillation of evidence and wisdom about audit presented in this book will help you to create audit programmes that are capable of bringing about real improvements.

The National Institute for Clinical Excellence and the Commission for Health Improvement will each have an important part to play in setting the national context within which the NHS addresses the need to review the quality of healthcare. But the real worth of clinical audit will depend on the commitment of local NHS staff and organisations. We hope that this book will help provide a framework for clinical audit that maximises local enthusiasm and commitment to high-quality patient care.

Dame Deirdre Hine
Chair
Commission for Health Improvement

Sir Michael Rawlins
Chairman
National Institute for Clinical Excellence

Clinical audit in the NHS: a statement from the National Institute for Clinical Excellence

The clinical audit challenge facing the NHS

The NHS needs to change its approach to clinical audit, and this book sets out the principles that should guide those changes.

There have been significant shifts in society's attitude to quality in healthcare over recent years, culminating in the introduction of clinical governance for the NHS. As part of local arrangements for clinical governance, all NHS organisations are required to have a comprehensive programme of quality improvement activity that includes clinicians participating fully in audit. Clinical audit is the component of clinical governance that offers the greatest potential to assess the quality of care routinely provided for NHS users – audit should therefore be at the very heart of clinical governance systems.

For clinical audit to become an important component of how we manage our health services a very real change needs to take place in the standing of audit programmes within the NHS. Audit can no longer be seen as a fringe activity for enthusiasts – within clinical governance, the NHS needs to make a commitment to support audit as a mainstream activity.

Issues needing attention

In this book the authors set out two key areas for attention if audit is to play a part in bringing about real improvements in quality of care. First, efforts must be made to ensure that the NHS **creates the local environment** for audit. Second, the NHS needs to make sure that it **uses audit methods** that are most likely to lead to audit projects that result in real improvements. Both areas deserve serious attention at all levels in the NHS – and audit programmes are unlikely to be successful if NHS staff find themselves struggling with audit in the absence of appropriate **methods** and a supportive **environment**.

A mixed record for audit

Clinical audit has a mixed history in the NHS, and for every success story there are just as many projects that have run into the ground without demonstrating any significant contribution to quality of services. Many of audit's early adopters have lost the enthusiasm they once had. This legacy needs to be addressed if individuals and teams are to re-engage their hearts and minds in clinical audit.

Many audit projects have floundered as a result of poor project design. Problems with clinical data have been particularly common. Data have often been of poor quality and inaccessible, or alternatively have been collected because of administrative convenience even where they are not accepted as relevant measures of clinical quality. In many cases the dataset has been simply too large to be workable within a busy clinical service weighed down with other priorities.

Many projects have been poorly managed, inadequately carried out, or both. Change in complex healthcare systems cannot be brought about simply by the analysis of data that indicate that care might be less than perfect. The management of change is often more challenging than the clinical issues addressed by audit, but all too often the change agenda has been left in the inexperienced hands of junior staff, without appropriate support.

Many projects that may have been well designed have taken place without any tangible senior support and commitment. This has made the conduct of audit an uphill struggle as enthusiastic teams find their ambitious plans thwarted by organisational inertia.

In many cases audit projects have failed to emphasise in their plans the need to devote just as much attention to changes that need to flow from audit as they have given to data collection and analysis. The failure to follow through audit towards improved practice has sometimes been the result of design problems, sometimes lack of senior support and commitment. In both cases healthcare staff rapidly lose their enthusiasm when they are unable to see benefit for their patients from the considerable extra commitment needed to mount a worthwhile audit project.

Despite this mixed record, there have been significant successes for clinical audit. Many local projects have provided a systematic structure through which clinical teams have been able to deliver real improvements in patient care. In some cases national projects have been able to play an important role in service-wide changes in care, bringing improved access and quality of care throughout the country (the national audit of stroke care is perhaps the most well known of these).

So recent experiences of clinical audit give good reason to believe that audit can be made to work – but the NHS must use well-founded **audit methods** within a supportive **environment**.

Clinical audit as part of professional accountability

Society has increasingly questioned quality of care and concepts of professional discretion or clinical freedom. The stark evidence of this shift in attitudes is shown in the demands of pressure groups, press coverage, calls for public inquiries, and the rise of complaints, legal challenges and claims for redress.

Yet patients and the public have not lost their respect and appreciation for the caring professions in the health service. Practitioners, patients, and the wider public all share equally in the need to establish and maintain confidence in the quality of clinical care. Audit is one way in which we can work to retain the trust and respect in an increasingly critical environment. As a quality improvement tool, audit can demonstrate that real efforts are being made by dedicated, hard-pressed staff to deliver high-quality professional care to all their patients.

Clinical audit is increasingly seen as an essential component of professional practice, and we welcome the emphasis professional bodies, regulators, and Government are giving to professional participation and leadership of audit.

The way forward

When done well, clinical audit has provided a way in which the quality of the care can be reviewed objectively, within an approach that is supportive and developmental. Changes in society have subjected all areas of professional practice to question and challenge. Clinical audit provides practitioners with a systematic response that compares the care provided to best practice while preserving the central role of the clinical team in agreeing and implementing plans for change.

Clinical governance presents a new challenge – to take audit 'at its best' and incorporate it within organisation-wide approaches to quality. We hope that this book will help NHS organisations **create the environment** and **use the methods** to support best practice in clinical audit throughout the NHS.

David Pink, Audit Programme Director
National Institute for Clinical Excellence
January 2002

Introduction: using the method, creating the environment

What is clinical audit?

Clinical audit is a quality improvement process that seeks to improve patient care and outcomes through systematic review of care against explicit criteria and the implementation of change. Aspects of the structure, processes, and outcomes of care are selected and systematically evaluated against explicit criteria. Where indicated, changes are implemented at an individual, team, or service level and further monitoring is used to confirm improvement in healthcare delivery.

This definition is endorsed by the National Institute for Clinical Excellence.

Who is this book for?

This book is written primarily for staff leading clinical audit and clinical governance projects and programmes in the NHS. It should also prove useful to many other people involved in audit projects, large or small and in primary or secondary care.

Why should I read it?

Every NHS health professional seeks to improve the quality of patient care. The concept that clinical audit can provide the framework in which this can be done collaboratively and systematically is reflected in current NHS policy statements.

- As a first step, clinical audit was integrated into clinical governance systems (Department of Health, 1997; Welsh Office, 1996).
- Full participation in clinical audit by all hospital doctors was subsequently made an explicit component of clinical governance (Department of Health, 1998; Welsh Office, 1998).

- *The NHS Plan* (Department of Health, 2000) has taken these policies further, with proposals for mandatory participation by all doctors in clinical audit and developments to support the involvement of other staff, including nurses, midwives, therapists and other NHS staff. *Improving Health in Wales* (Minister for Health and Social Services, 2001) introduced annual appraisals that address the results of audit.

The General Medical Council now advises all doctors that they: 'must take part in regular and systematic medical and clinical audit, recording data honestly. Where necessary, you must respond to the results of audit to improve your practice, for example by undertaking further training' (General Medical Council, 2001). The UK Central Council for Nursing, Midwifery and Health Visiting states that clinical governance, assisting the coordination of quality improvement initiatives such as clinical audit, is: 'the business of every registered practitioner' (UK Central Council for Nursing, Midwifery and Health Visiting, 2001).

The recommendations of *Learning from Bristol: the Report of the Public Inquiry into Children's Heart Surgery at the Bristol Royal Infirmary 1984–1995* (Department of Health, 2001) (referred to hereafter as 'the Bristol Royal Infirmary Inquiry') can now be added to these statements. In particular, the Inquiry makes the following recommendations.

143 The process of clinical audit, which is now widely practised within trusts, should be at the core of a system of local monitoring of performance.

144 Clinical audit must be fully supported by trusts. They should ensure that healthcare professionals have access to the necessary time, facilities, advice, and expertise in order to conduct audit effectively. All trusts should have a central clinical audit office that coordinates audit activity, provides advice and support for the audit process, and brings together the results of audit for the trust as a whole.

145 Clinical audit should be compulsory for all healthcare professionals providing clinical care and the requirement to participate in it should be included as part of the contract of employment.

The Government has welcomed the recommendations of the Bristol Royal Infirmary Inquiry (*Learning from Bristol: the Department of Health's Response to the Report of the Public Inquiry into Children's Heart Surgery at the Bristol Royal Infirmary 1984–1995*, 2002) (the full set of recommendations relevant to audit and the Government's response are to be found at Appendix VIII.)

It follows that all healthcare professionals need to understand the principles of clinical audit, and the organisations in which they work must support them in undertaking clinical audit.

Using the method

Clinical audit can be described as a cycle or a spiral (*see* Figure 1). Within the cycle there are stages that follow a systematic process of establishing best practice,

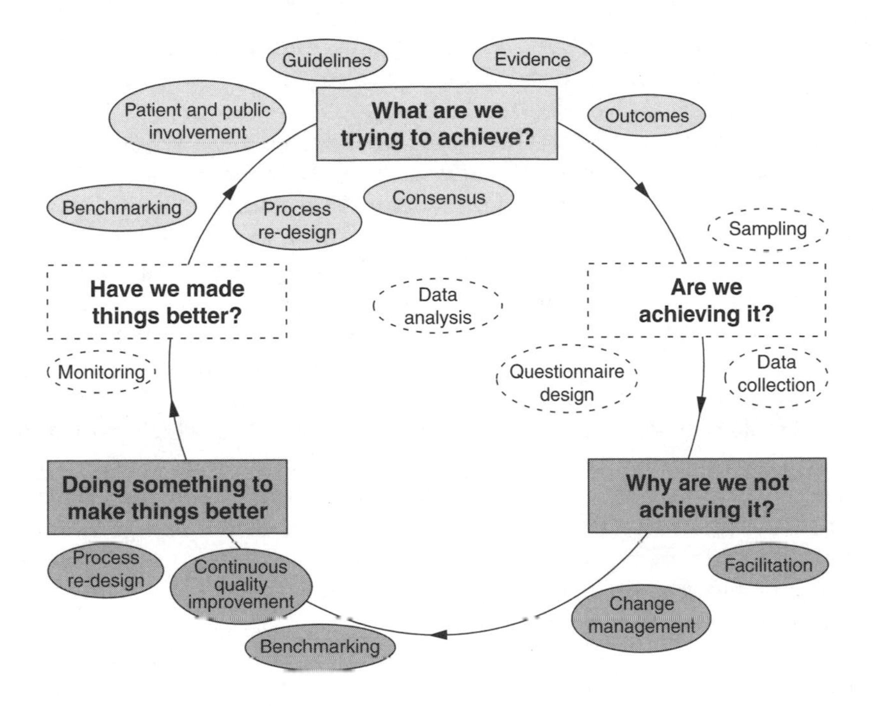

Figure 1. The clinical audit cycle.

measuring care against criteria, taking action to improve care, and monitoring to sustain improvement. The spiral suggests that as the process continues, each cycle aspires to a higher level of quality.

Clinical audit requires the use of a broad range of methods from a number of disciplines, for example, organisational development, statistics, and information management. Clinical audit can be undertaken by individual healthcare staff, or groups of professionals in single or multidisciplinary teams, usually supported by clinical audit staff from NHS trusts or primary care organisations. At the opposite end of the scale, a clinical audit project may involve all services in a region or even in the country. Effective systems for managing the audit project and implementing change are important whether a large number of people or only a few are involved in the audit project. At the start of an audit project, spending time on creating the right environment may be more important than spending time on the method itself.

Creating the environment

The Government has introduced clinical governance to support organisational change in the way care is delivered within the NHS. Clinical governance has been defined as: '. . . a framework through which NHS organisations are accountable for continuously improving the quality of their services and safeguarding high standards of care by creating an environment in which excellence in clinical care will flourish' (Department of Health, 1998; Welsh Office, 1998).

For clinical governance to fulfil its promise, new skills are required, including improved understanding of clinical audit and of the need for an organisational environment that supports effective clinical audit. The evidence for this is presented in the literature review, which is enclosed with this book as a CD-ROM. The review without the evidence tables is also included in Appendix XI. If the organisational environment is supportive, the staff involved are well prepared and the methods fully understood, clinical audit has every chance of succeeding. Where audit methodology is poorly understood, or the organisational environment is not supportive, there is less chance of clinical audit being successful.

The methodology of clinical audit and the environment in which it operates are interrelated. If the environment is supportive but clinical audit methods are not used appropriately, there may be less improvement than expected, or no evidence that improvements have been made. Similarly, if clinical audit methods are used well but in an environment that is not supportive, the result may also be a failure to improve care and frustration among those involved.

The environment can be divided into:

- structure
- culture.

The structure provides a practical link between the business of clinical governance, professional self-regulation, and lifelong learning. It is a key task for those charged with leading health service organisations to provide the necessary structure, for example facilities like time, technical support, or library services. Facilities alone are not enough, however: a culture is required in which creativity and openness are encouraged, and errors and failures are reported and investigated without fear of blame.

How to use this book

The main text of this book is divided into five chapters, each addressing one of the five stages of clinical audit (*see* Figure 2). In the chapters we, the authors, draw on our review of the recent literature on clinical audit to describe the methods, tools, techniques, and activities related to each stage. Although the methods provide the focus for each chapter, the parallel message that the environment must support each stage runs throughout, and is dealt with in more detail in Stage Five. Referencing has been kept minimal in the main text chapters to avoid distracting the reader and the full reference list supporting the literature review can be found in Appendix XI.

The evidence described in the literature review shows that much has been learned about audit in recent years. It is now time to build on this experience by designing, undertaking and implementing successful clinical audit projects.

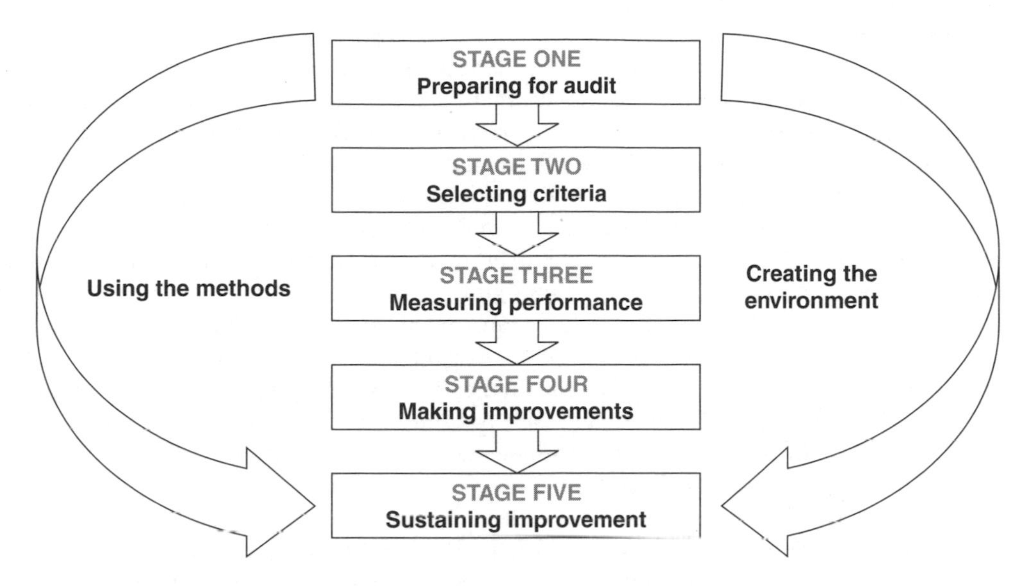

Figure 2. The stages of clinical audit. Clinical audit involves the use of specific methods, but also requires the creation of a supportive environment.

The review of the evidence is an update of *Good Practice in Clinical Audit: a Summary of Selected Literature to Support Criteria for Clinical Audit*, published by the National Centre for Clinical Audit (Dixon, 1996).

Key points

From the review of the literature, we identified a set of key points for best practice in clinical audit. These are included at the start of the relevant chapters, and the full set is included as an appendix. The key points relate directly to the literature review so, if you want to explore a key point in greater depth, you can refer to the related evidence in the review (either in Appendix XI or the CD-ROM which includes all the tables).

Key notes

In addition to the key points, the book discusses a number of issues that are not addressed in the reviewed literature, or for which evidence is limited. These are the 'key notes', and again these are presented at the start of the relevant chapters, with a full set supplied as an appendix.

Appendices

A number of appendices are included as additional resources/reference material to help plan local audit programmes. They include: a glossary explaining terminology;

a guide to online resources for clinical audit; a list of national audit projects, sponsored by the National Institute for Clinical Excellence; recommendations from the Bristol Royal Infirmary Inquiry and the Government's response; lessons learnt from the National Sentinel Audit Programme; information from the Commission for Health Improvement on examining clinical audit during a clinical governance review; a list of the desirable characteristics of audit review criteria; and a further reading list.

Also included are checklists developed from the key points and key notes from each stage. These are designed to complement other assessment tools, summarising the important elements of clinical audit highlighted within the book. Reviewing audit projects, or plans for projects, can help to improve their quality, and these checklists can aid the design and conduct of audits. They can be used by clinicians or audit staff before an audit starts, or after it has finished to look at what might have been done differently. A checklist for reviewing audit programmes is also included, and those who lead audit in health service organisations may use it to identify ways in which their programmes could be strengthened.

Although the checklists are intended as learning aids, they are not suited to use as part of a formal assessment process, for which other audit review systems are available. The Commission for Health Improvement (CHI) assesses audit programmes as part of its reviews of health service organisations (the key elements included in the CHI review are described in an appendix). A particularly useful review system for trusts enables self-assessment of the performance of the audit programme and can be used to complement the checklists in this book (Walshe and Spurgeon, 1997); this can be downloaded from www.hsmc3.bham.ac.uk/hsmc.

The findings of the literature review are set out in Appendix XI.

Electronic access

All the resources associated with this book and the full literature review are available on the CD-ROM and via the NICE website (www.nice.org.uk).

References

Department of Health. *The New NHS: Modern, Dependable*. London: The Stationery Office, 1997.

Department of Health. *A First Class Service. Quality in the New NHS*. London: Department of Health, 1998.

Department of Health. *The NHS Plan: A Plan for Investment – A Plan for Reform*. London: The Stationery Office, 2000.

Department of Health. *Learning from Bristol: the Report of the Public Inquiry into Children's Heart Surgery at the Bristol Royal Infirmary 1984–1995*. Command paper CM 5207. London: The Stationery Office, 2001.

Department of Health. *Learning from Bristol: the Department of Health's Response to the Report of the Public Inquiry into Children's Heart Surgery at the Bristol Royal Infirmary 1984–1995*. Command paper CM 5363. London: The Stationery Office, 2002.

Dixon N. *Good Practice in Clinical Audit – A Summary of Selected Literature to Support Criteria for Clinical Audit*. London: National Centre for Clinical Audit, 1996.

General Medical Council. *Good Medical Practice*. London: General Medical Council, 2001.

Minister for Health and Social Services. *Improving Health in Wales – A Plan for the NHS and its Partners*. Cardiff: National Assembly for Wales, 2001.

UK Central Council for Nursing, Midwifery and Health Visiting. *Professional Self-Regulation and Clinical Governance*. London: United Kingdom Central Council for Nursing, Midwifery and Health Visiting, 2001.

Walshe K, Spurgeon P. *Clinical Audit Assessment Framework. HSMC Handbook Series 24*. Birmingham: University of Birmingham, 1997.

Welsh Office. *Framework for the Development of Multi-professional Clinical Audit*. Cardiff: Welsh Office, 1996.

Welsh Office. *Quality Care and Clinical Excellence*. Cardiff: Welsh Office, 1998.

Stage One: preparing for audit

Key points

- Clinical audit is used to improve aspects of care in a wide variety of topics. It is also used in association with changes in systems of care, or to confirm that current practice meets the expected level of performance.
- Clinical audit projects are best conducted within a structured programme, with effective leadership, participation by all staff, and an emphasis on team working and support.
- Organisations must recognise that clinical audit requires appropriate funding.
- Organisations need to recognise that improvements in care resulting from clinical audit can increase costs.
- The participation of staff in selecting topics enables concerns about care to be reported and addressed. Participation in choice of topic is not always necessary, but may have a role in reducing resistance to change.
- The priorities of those receiving care can differ quite markedly from those of clinicians. Service users should therefore be involved in the clinical audit process.
- There are practical approaches for user involvement in all stages of audit, including the design, the collection of data about performance, and in implementing change.
- Organisations should ensure that their healthcare staff learn the skills of clinical audit.
- The most frequently cited barrier to successful clinical audit is the failure of organisations to provide sufficient protected time for healthcare teams.
- Those involved in organising audit programmes must consider various methods of engaging the full participation of all health service staff.

Good preparation is crucial to the success of an audit project. National audit projects reviewed by the National Institute for Clinical Excellence (NICE) suggest that two broad areas of preparation must be addressed (*see* Appendix IX):

- project management, including topic selection, planning and resources, and communication
- project methodology, including design, data issues, implementability, stakeholder involvement, and the provision of support for local improvement.

In practical terms, preparing for audit can be broken down into five elements that are discussed through the chapter:

- involving users in the process (for the purpose of this book, the terms 'users' and 'service users' include patients, other service users and carers, and members of groups and organisations that represent their interests)
- topic selection
- defining the purpose of the audit
- providing the necessary structures
- identifying the skills and people needed to carry out the audit, and training staff and encouraging them to participate.

An example of the factors that contributed to a successful audit (in secondary care) is shown in Table 1.

Table 1. An example of factors contributing to the success of an audit (secondary care). The audit took place in a Walsall clinic for survivors of myocardial infarction; coronary heart disease is a major health issue in Walsall (Giles *et al.*, 1998)

- Support from the health authority
- Partnership with primary care
- A good link with the patient support group
- Involvement of patients
- A good evidence base for guidelines
- Effective distribution of guidelines
- Use of information technology
- Improved record keeping
- Audit used as an inbuilt element of work

Involving users

The focus of any audit project must be those receiving care. Users can be genuine collaborators, rather than merely sources of data (Balogh *et al.*, 1995).

Sources of user information

The concerns of users can be identified from various sources, including:

- letters containing comments or complaints
- critical incident reports
- individual patients' stories or feedback from focus groups
- direct observation of care
- direct conversations.

The most common method of involving users in clinical audit is the satisfaction survey. Involvement of users in the planning and negotiation of topics for audit is much less common. Some sources of guidance on how to involve users and the public at different stages of the audit cycle are given in Appendix IV.

New systems for user involvement

Systems are being introduced into the NHS locally to identify and discuss the issues that are of most concern to service users; for example, in England, each trust will have a Patient Forum and a Patient Advocacy and Liaison Service (Department of Health, 2000). These systems are not focused on audit, but they will provide a route through which topics for audit can be identified. Trusts will also be required to undertake regular user surveys.

The involvement of users in decisions about their health is also central to the new direction in health and social policy in Wales (Minister for Health and Social Services, 2001). For example, in Wales:

- Local Health Groups and NHS trusts produce public involvement plans
- 'signpost' guidance has been issued to the NHS to assist preparation of baseline assessments of public involvement
- Community Health Councils have been retained and strengthened to ensure the most effective representation of patients.

The publication *A Guide to Involving Older People in Local Clinical Audit Activity: National Sentinel Audits Involving Older People* (Kelson, 1999) offers practical advice and many examples of how older people can assist at many stages of the audit cycle, from selection of topics to dissemination of findings. One example is a project in Fife, in which user panels consisting of housebound people over 75 years of age contributed to the development of a hospital discharge policy. In a project to involve patients with brain tumours in an assessment of the service at King's College Hospital, London, a process map of the patient's journey through the service was developed and randomly selected patients were interviewed in their own homes (Grimes, 2000). After analysing patients' comments and identifying problems, new documentation was produced to help staff through issues requiring discussion with patients during their stay in hospital. Aspects of outpatient activity, such as turn-around times for biopsy results and availability of clinical scans, were also addressed.

National involvement

At a national level, there is a responsibility to ensure that clinical audit is an integral part of the quality improvement and clinical governance strategies. NICE provides guidance on clinical audit with its guidelines, and as part of its clinical governance reviews the Commission for Health Improvement (CHI) ensures that NHS trusts and primary care organisations undertake audit. CHI's reports give a detailed assessment of the state of clinical audit within an organisation, citing examples of good and poor practice (Table 2). Further details of the review process and clinical governance reports are available from CHI's website (www.chi.nhs.uk). In addition, the Royal Colleges and professional bodies are involved, with their members, in raising awareness and support for clinical audit.

Table 2. Poor practice identified in one trust during a clinical governance review carried out by the CHI. The trust was urged to make greater use of clinical audit to improve services for users, encourage multidisciplinary audits, and ensure that findings were implemented, monitored, and evaluated

- Clinical audits in response to reported incidents, complaints, NICE guidance or National Service Frameworks were seldom performed
- Few multidisciplinary audits were undertaken
- Patients' perspectives were not generally considered
- There was no systematic implementation or follow-up of audit findings, despite examples of good practice in some directorates

Users in audit projects teams

Users are increasingly involved as members of clinical audit project teams. Where users are involved in this way, careful thought needs to be given to issues of access, preparation and support (Kelson, 1998).

Selecting a topic

The starting point for many quality improvement initiatives – selecting a topic for audit – needs careful thought and planning, because any clinical audit project needs a significant investment of resources.

Audit priorities

The clinical team has an important role in prioritising clinical topics, and the following questions may be a useful discussion guide.

- Is the topic concerned of high cost, volume, or risk to staff or users?
- Is there evidence of a serious quality problem, for example patient complaints or high complication rates?
- Is good evidence available to inform standards, for example systematic reviews or national clinical guidelines?
- Is the problem concerned amenable to change?
- Is there potential for involvement in a national audit project?
- Is the topic pertinent to national policy initiatives?
- Is the topic a priority for the organisation?

Each healthcare organisation has its own priorities for clinical audit. For example, in many NHS organisations a committee or clinical effectiveness/governance team decides which clinical audit projects should be undertaken in any particular year. Their decisions are usually based on local health priorities, which reflect national targets, for example in cancer services, coronary care, or mental health. Projects may also need to focus on the implementation of National Service Frameworks, Health Improvement Plans, or NICE guidelines and appraisals.

Some issues may also become important because of the need for public accountability. An example of this is a recent project led by the Royal College of Psychiatrists, which used a postal survey of 1700 people who used, provided, or purchased mental health services to identify the topic regarded as having the highest priority for improvement. The results of the survey led to the development of guidelines and clinical audit on the management of imminent violence (www.psychiatry.ox.ac.uk/cebmh/guidelines).

Some projects may benefit from being associated with specialty audits conducted by Royal Colleges or professional bodies, or with regional projects, clinical practice benchmarking initiatives, or national audits.

When all the various sources have been considered, the topics suggested need to be prioritised in a systematic way. It is important to ensure that the views of users, clinical staff, support staff, and managers are represented in the selection process. A scoring system could help to rank topics in order of importance, such as quality impact analysis or a locally developed grid listing the selection criteria and ranking topics accordingly.

Defining the purpose

A project without clear objectives cannot achieve anything: a clear sense of purpose must be established before appropriate methods for audit can be considered. Once the topic for a clinical audit project has been selected, therefore, the purpose of the project must be defined, so that a suitable audit method can be chosen. The following series of verbs may be useful in defining the aims of an audit (Buttery, 1998):

- to improve
- to enhance

- to ensure
- to change.

Examples of using these are:

- to improve the blood transfusion processes within the trust
- to increase the proportion of patients with hypertension whose blood pressure is controlled
- to ensure that every infant has access to immunisation against diphtheria, tetanus, pertussis, polio, influenza B, and meningitis C before 6 months of age.

During the planning stage of an audit, it is important to consider the mechanisms for project management. The audit methods, including the aims and objectives, criteria and target levels of performance, data requirements, data collection instrument, and agreed terms, should all be documented. Ideally, these components should be collated into a project record that will evolve according to the stages of the project, and be updated at each project milestone. In this way, the project record can progress from an initial proposal to a final report of the audit outcome.

Providing a structure

To enhance the benefits of audit, an organisation needs:

- a structured audit programme (committee structure, feedback mechanisms, regular audit meetings)
- a team of well-qualified audit staff (Dickinson and Edwards, 1999).

Quality assurance

Each NHS organisation is responsible for assuring the quality of clinical audit, which is discussed in more detail in Stage Five: sustaining improvement. A project assessment framework can be used for reviewing clinical audit. One proposed framework includes nine elements (reasons for topic selection, impact, costs, objectives, involvement, use of evidence, project management, methods, and evaluation) (Walshe and Spurgeon, 1997), but does not include the ethical issues associated with audit, though these should be taken into account (*see* Stage Three: measuring level of performance). Such ethical issues include consent, confidentiality, effectiveness of audit, and accountability (Morrell and Harvey, 1999).

Funding

Support for clinical audit includes the provision of funding for audit, and the appropriate use of funds when responding to the findings of audit. The cost of clinical audit staff with the breadth of skills to work across the range of issues encompassed within clinical governance is significant. Clinical staff will struggle to complete effective clinical audit projects unless they have expert support in terms of project management, knowledge of clinical audit techniques, facilitation, data management, staff training and administration. Funding is also required for clinical staff to participate in audit (*see* Stage Two: selecting criteria).

Clinical audit projects are expensive and their costs must be justifiable. Project assessments should include cost as part of the review (Walshe and Spurgeon, 1997). It should be remembered, however, that the topics selected for clinical audit are priorities within a given service, and the clinical audit process can provide valuable data to assist decision-making about the use of resources locally within that service. Budget holders must seriously consider any findings that a service needs further resources in order to improve.

One example of this is an audit project undertaken to identify all patients taking angiotensin-converting enzyme (ACE) inhibitors in one general practice, focusing on those whose blood pressure was not maintained below 160/90 mmHg. The impact of various interventions on the cost of improving care was analysed at the end of the audit cycle. The audit showed that it was possible to reduce blood pressure further in a significant number of patients receiving ACE inhibitors, but drug costs and the number of referrals to specialist services would both rise (Jiwa and Mathers, 2000).

Making time

The main barriers to audit reported in the literature are lack of resources, especially time. Both protected time to investigate the audit topic and collect and analyse data, and time to complete an audit cycle are in short supply. Clearly, if clinical audit is to fulfil its potential as a model for quality improvement, staff of all grades need to be allocated the time to participate fully.

Identifying and developing skills for audit projects

To be successful, a clinical audit project needs to involve the right people with the right skills from the outset. Therefore, identifying the skills required and organising the key individuals should be priorities.

Certain skills are needed for all audit projects, and these include:

- project leadership, project organisation, project management
- clinical, managerial, and other service input and leadership
- audit method expertise
- change management skills
- data collection and data analysis skills
- facilitation skills.

Audit project teams

The usual approach, even for small projects, is to set up an audit project team customised to the specific audit project, with team members providing many of the skills needed. For example, clinical service representatives and audit staff are usually included in audit project teams. It is also important that the team includes members from all the relevant groups involved in care delivery, and not just those with clinical experience. So, according to the project topic, an audit project team in a primary care setting may include a surgery receptionist, while a team in secondary care may include porters or catering staff. All audit projects need direct access to people with a full understanding of the processes of clinical care and the information systems used within the service, and this essential real-world knowledge is most likely to be found from the staff working in the service.

All project team members should have:

- a basic understanding of clinical audit (one barrier to successful audit highlighted in the review of the evidence is lack of training and audit skills)
- an understanding of and commitment to the plans and objectives of the project
- an understanding of what is expected of the project team – this needs to be clarified at the outset and may be expressed in a 'terms of reference' document.

It may also be useful to establish ground rules for meetings, so that everyone is clear about the way in which the team will function. A trained facilitator can guide and enable effective team working.

Finally, if the audit team is to improve the performance of a clinical service, team members must be able to communicate effectively with their colleagues. Members of the project team must, therefore, have the full confidence and support of the staff and organisation and be able to promote the audit and plans for quality improvement.

Role of clinical audit staff in audit projects

A good understanding of audit methods, as well as significant organisational and analytical skills, is needed when carrying out many clinical audits. Local audit staff can provide expert help.

Clinical audit staff have a number of important roles, though these may differ between organisations.

- **Information/knowledge support** – in collaboration with colleagues in library and information services, audit teams should have access to information technology (IT) facilities to help gather evidence for standard setting and search for other projects on the same topic.
- **Data management** – clinical audit staff have expertise in data collection, entry, analysis, and presentation.
- **Facilitation** – some clinical audit staff have particular training and skills in group dynamics. The role of a facilitator in the context of clinical audit is to help the team

to assimilate the evidence, to come to a common understanding of the clinical audit methodology, to guide the project from planning to reporting, and to enable the group to work together effectively.

- **Project management** – project management and leadership is an important factor in quality improvement projects. In the words of McCrea (1999), 'Since both health care and clinical audit depend on the quality of teamwork, more attention needs to be given to the development of appropriate skills of team leadership.' Achieving improvements in quality through clinical audit often depends on managing relationships and resources across the wider organisation as well as addressing issues within the team immediately involved in the audit.
- **Training** – in many NHS organisations, audit staff are involved in training and support on a wide range of quality improvements skills for clinicians, managers and others involved in clinical governance.

Healthcare Quality Quest (1999) and the Clinical Audit Association (www.the-caa-ltd.demon.co.uk) have developed organisational roles and competencies related to clinical effectiveness and clinical audit to make explicit the way in which designated audit staff and clinical staff work together to improve the quality of care.

Developing skills

Lack of training and audit skills is highlighted in the review of the evidence as a barrier to successful audit. One assessment framework states that an ongoing programme of training in clinical audit for clinical professionals should be available to members of clinical staff from different departments/services and different professions (Walshe and Spurgeon, 1997). Advice and support for clinical audit are, in fact, available to staff working in most NHS organisations, and may include:

- advice, including the selection of methods
- ongoing help in the use of methods
- access to training in clinical audit methods.

Although many NHS trusts and primary care organisations run excellent 'in-house' clinical audit training, staff are often unable to attend because of their other duties. Providing sufficient cover for staff development and training has budgetary implications – indeed, staff salaries are the major expense involved in clinical audit. This is a key issue in developing organisational strategies to support clinical governance, and needs to be taken seriously if clinical audit is to be successful.

Encouraging and supporting staff participation in audit

In any clinical audit project, the people involved in delivering and receiving care should be involved, either directly or by means of representation, from start to finish.

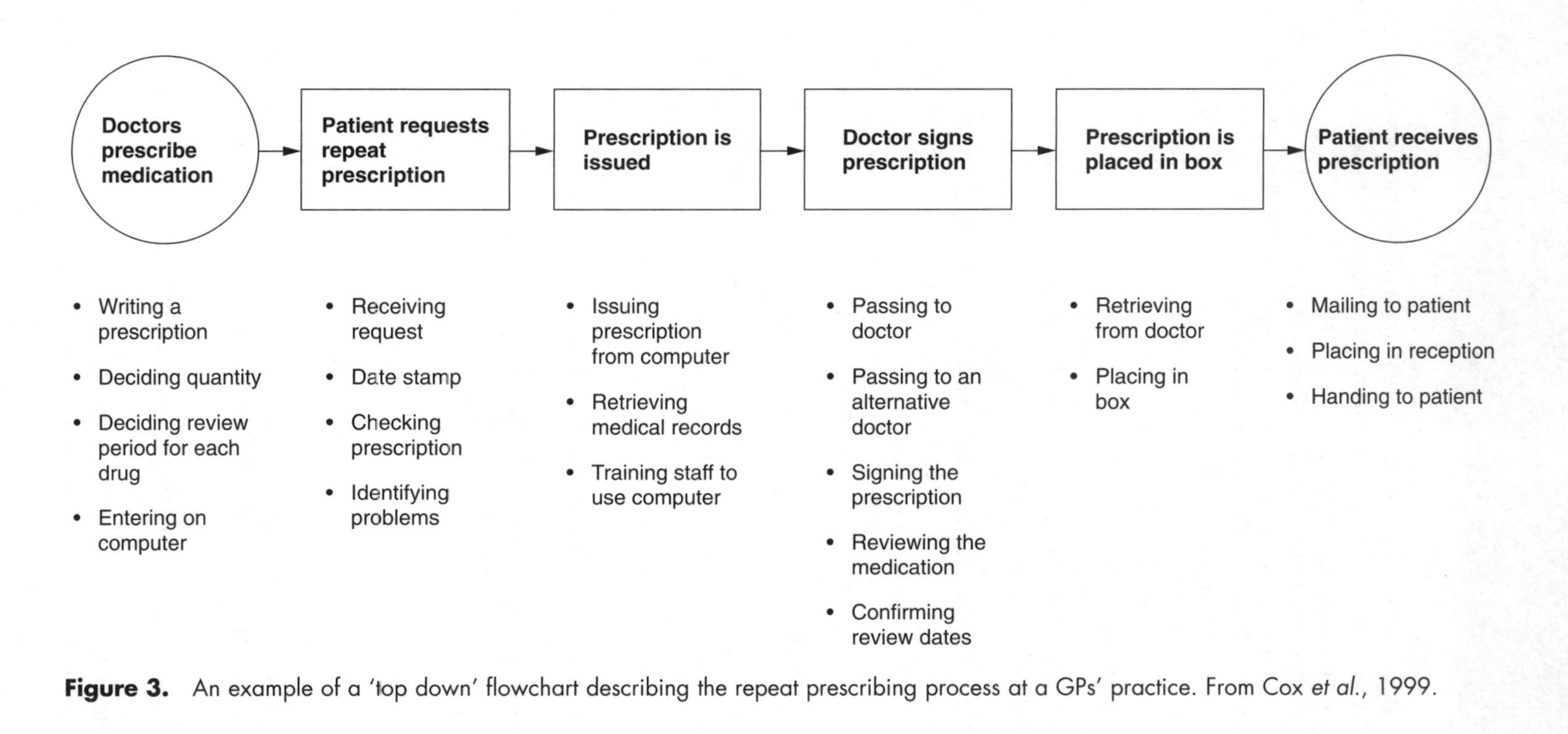

Figure 3. An example of a 'top down' flowchart describing the repeat prescribing process at a GPs' practice. From Cox *et al.*, 1999.

By showing individuals the relevance of involvement in clinical audit to their personal development and re-accreditation, clinical activities take on a new meaning within a clinical governance framework (Houghton *et al.*, 1999). A facilitator can play a central role in gaining the participation of all who should be involved.

Drawing a flowchart to illustrate the major steps and activities undertaken within the care process is a helpful way of identifying the people who should be involved in an audit (an example is shown in Figure 3). Flowcharting, or work flow analysis as it is sometimes called, helps teams to:

- explore the relationships between different activities
- identify stakeholders (those who will be affected by the audit)
- focus attention on where improvement efforts need to be concentrated.

It also reflects the key features of systems that contribute to errors occurring.

The involvement of healthcare staff in audit can be secured in two main ways.

- Firstly, appropriate strategies are used to ensure that staff regard clinical audit and data collection as an integral part of their job (Schein, 1997). Referring to audit in the recruitment and selection process, including it in job descriptions, discussing it in appraisal interviews, and providing information about the organisation's audit programme are all potential strategies for this embedding process.
- Secondly, systems to encourage active involvement are devised, so that the process is owned by those carrying out the audit rather than being imposed from above (Bate, 1998). The process of selecting topics for audit offers an obvious opportunity to involve a range of healthcare staff and service users.

The degree of involvement of managers in clinical audit projects will vary, but a lack of commitment from managers can lead to serious misunderstandings. So, it is vital that all managers understand the aims of audit and support those involved.

Understanding audit

Everyone who becomes involved in an audit project needs an understanding of audit in general and the objectives of the project. The wider staff to be involved in the audit may have development needs, in addition to those of the audit team (*see* 'Developing skills' on page 17). The adoption of a common language is particularly important, as inconsistent terminology can create problems for staff with different professional or academic backgrounds. For example, the terms 'standard' and 'criterion' may be interpreted differently by staff with different backgrounds (these particular terms are discussed in Stage Two: selecting criteria).

References

Balogh R, Simpson A, Bond S. Involving clients in clinical audits of mental health services. *International Journal for Quality in Health Care* 1995; 7: 343–53.

Bate SP. *Strategies for Cultural Change*. Oxford: Butterworth-Heinemann, 1998.

Buttery Y. Implementing evidence through clinical audit. In: *Evidence-based Healthcare*. Oxford: Butterworth-Heinemann, 1998: 182–207.

Cox S, Wilcock P, Young J. Improving the repeat prescribing process in a busy general practice. A study using continuous quality improvement methodology. *Quality in Health Care* 1999; **8**: 119–125.

Department of Health. *The NHS Plan: A Plan for Investment – A Plan for Reform*. London: The Stationery Office, 2000.

Dickinson K, Edwards J. Clinical audit: failure or hidden success? *Journal of Clinical Excellence* 1999; **1**: 97–100.

Giles PD, Cunnington AR, Payne M, Crothers DC, Walsh MS. Cholesterol reduction for the secondary prevention of coronary heart disease: a successful multi-disciplinary approach to implementing evidence-based treatment in a district general hospital. *Journal of Clinical Effectiveness* 1998; **3**: 156–60.

Grimes K. Using patients' views to improve a health care service. *Journal of Clinical Excellence* 2000; 2: 99–102.

Healthcare Quality Quest. *Clinical Audit Manual: Using Clinical Audit to Improve Clinical Effectiveness*. Romsey: Healthcare Quality Quest, 1999.

Houghton G, O'Mahoney D, Sturman SG, Unsworth J. The clinical implementation of clinical governance: acute stroke management as an example. *Journal of Clinical Excellence* 1999; **1**: 129–32.

Jiwa M, Mathers N. Auditing the use of ACE inhibitors in hypertension. Reflecting the cost of clinical governance? *Journal of Clinical Governance* 2000; **8**: 27–30.

Kelson M. *Promoting Patient Involvement in Clinical Audit: Practical Guidance on Achieving Effective Involvement*. London: College of Health, 1998.

Kelson M. *A Guide to Involving Older People in Local Clinical Audit Activity: National Sentinel Audits Involving Older People*. London: College of Health, 1999.

McCrea C. Good clinical audit requires teamwork. In: Baker R, Hearnshaw H, Robertson N, eds. *Implementing Change with Clinical Audit*. Chichester: Wiley, 1999: 119–32.

Minister for Health and Social Services. *Improving Health in Wales – A Plan for the NHS and its Partners*. Cardiff: National Assembly for Wales, 2001.

Morrell C, Harvey G. *The Clinical Audit Handbook*. London: Baillière Tindall, 1999.

Schein EH. *Organizational Culture and Leadership*. 2nd edition. San Francisco: Jossey Bass, 1997.

Walshe K, Spurgeon P. *Clinical Audit Assessment Framework, HSMC Handbook Series 24*. Birmingham: University of Birmingham, 1997.

Stage Two: selecting criteria

Key points

- Clinical audit can include assessment of the process and/or outcome of care. The choice depends on the topic and objectives of the audit.
- Explicit rather than implicit criteria should be preferred.
- Systematic methods should be used to derive criteria from evidence. These include methods for deriving criteria from good-quality guidelines or from reviews of the evidence.
- Criteria should relate to important aspects of care and be measurable.
- Provided that research evidence confirms that clinical care processes have an influence on outcome, measurement of the process of care is generally more sensitive and provides a direct measure of the quality of care.
- Measurement of outcome can be used to identify problems in care, provided outcomes are clear, influenced by process, and occur within a short period.
- Adjustment for case mix is generally required for comparing the outcomes of different providers.
- If the criteria incorporate, or are based on, the views of professionals or other groups, formal consensus methods are preferable.
- There is insufficient evidence to determine whether it is necessary to set target levels of performance in audit. However, reference to levels achieved in audits undertaken by other professionals is useful.
- In some audits, benchmarking techniques could help participants in audit to avoid setting unnecessarily low or unrealistically high target levels of performance.

Defining criteria

Within clinical audit, criteria are used to assess the quality of care provided by an individual, a team, or an organisation. These criteria:

- are explicit statements that define what is being measured
- represent elements of care that can be measured objectively.

Recent Government publications indicate that health professionals will be expected to develop criteria and standards that measure a wide range of features of quality in healthcare, such as access to care as well as satisfaction with the care received (Department of Health, 2000).

Different professional groups have used different definitions of 'criteria' and 'standards' (Tables 3 and 4). For clarity, this book uses the definition of criteria from the Institute of Medicine and the phrase 'level of performance' rather than the potentially more confusing term 'standard'.

Table 3. Definitions of a 'criterion'

- An item or variable which enables the achievement of a standard (broad objective of care) and the evaluation of whether it has been achieved or not (Royal College of Nursing, 1990)
- A definable and measurable item of healthcare which describes quality and which can be used to assess it (Irvine and Irvine, 1991)
- A systematically developed statement that can be used to assess the appropriateness of specific healthcare decisions, services, and outcomes (Institute of Medicine, 1992)

Table 4. Definitions of a 'standard'

- An objective with guidance for its achievement given in the form of criteria sets which specify required resources, activities, and predicted outcomes (Royal College of Nursing, 1990)
- The level of care to be achieved for any particular criterion (Irvine and Irvine, 1991)
- The percentage of events that should comply with the criterion (Baker and Fraser, 1995)

Criteria can be classified into those concerned with:

- structure (what you need)
- process (what you do)
- outcome of care (what you expect).

The advantage of categorising the criteria in this way is that if an outcome is not achieved and the structure and processes necessary have already been identified, the source of the problem should be easier to identify.

Structure criteria

Structure criteria refer to the resources required. They may include the numbers of staff and skill mix, organisational arrangements, the provision of equipment and physical space.

Process criteria

Process criteria refer to the actions and decisions taken by practitioners together with users. These actions may include communication, assessment, education, investigations, prescribing, surgical and other therapeutic interventions, evaluation, and documentation.

It has been argued that using process criteria encourages clinical teams to concentrate on the things they do that contribute directly to improved health outcomes. Process criteria are also more sensitive measures of the quality of care, as a poor outcome does not occur every time there is an error or omission in the provision of care. However, the importance of process criteria is determined by the extent to which they influence outcome.

Outcome criteria

Outcome criteria are typically measures of the physical or behavioural response to an intervention, reported health status, and level of knowledge and satisfaction. Sometimes surrogate, proxy, or intermediate outcome criteria are used instead. These relate to aspects of care that are closely linked to eventual outcome, but are more easily measured. For example, the intermediate outcome of blood pressure control in people with hypertension is a more practical and immediate measure for guiding improvements in care than eventual morbidity due to associated conditions.

Some audits focus specifically on outcomes and do not include formal criteria, but instead collect data about the outcomes of care. This is a practical possibility when outcomes are easily measurable and occur soon after the delivery of care. If the outcomes are also of major importance to users, for example postoperative complications, the direct measurement of outcome is not only appropriate but also expected. However, audit using outcome measures alone sometimes provides insufficient information for developing an action plan for improving practice.

When outcomes are used for comparative audit, adjustments may be needed for case mix, a process known as 'risk adjustment'. Failure to use either a formal or informal method of risk adjustment to account for any variation in patient populations sometimes leads to misinterpretation of the findings. However, it is important to avoid falling into the trap of assuming that poor outcomes are explained by case mix alone, when in fact they are due to failures in the process of care.

Developing valid criteria

Once a topic has been chosen, valid criteria must be selected. For criteria to be valid and lead to improvements in care, they need to be:

- based on evidence
- related to important aspects of care
- measurable.

Developing such criteria can be time-consuming and requires considerable expertise. An alternative is to use criteria developed by people who are trained in the processes of evaluating evidence from the literature and grading criteria by strength of evidence.

None of the methods of defining appropriate criteria is universally accepted. An international panel of experts has generated a set of desirable attributes of quality criteria, ranked by importance and feasibility (Hearnshaw *et al.*, 2001), and these are listed in Appendix X. This will form the starting point for work on an instrument for appraising the quality of criteria with the aim of improving the standard of quality improvement reviews, and hence, the quality of care.

Implicit criteria

In some situations, implicit criteria have been used (Dixon, 1996). This means that the review of care is undertaken by senior clinicians who rely on their own experience in judging care (Kahn *et al.*, 1989). For example, implicit criteria might be used in a case-note review of patients who have experienced adverse outcomes. Because of the difficulties of ensuring reliability in the interpretation of information about the care that was given, this method should be avoided where possible.

Using guidelines

Recommendations from clinical practice guidelines can be used to develop criteria and standards without substantial additional work. Guidelines now often include suggestions for criteria, a policy that will be followed in guidelines published by NICE. As the development of good-quality guidelines depends on careful review of the relevant research evidence, the criteria suggested in such guidelines are likely to be valid.

For example, the Scottish Intercollegiate Guidelines Network (SIGN) guideline on the secondary prevention of coronary heart disease following myocardial infarction (Scottish Intercollegiate Guidelines Network, 2000) lists several key points, including the prescribing of prophylactic medication, that could be used as the starting point for developing criteria for different subgroups of users (e.g. those being discharged from hospital following an infarct, or those under long-term care by general practitioners).

Criteria for the audit of treatment of the major diseases can also be developed directly from a literature search of specific journal articles, or from good-quality systematic reviews. There is no need to duplicate detailed literature searches, provided that an up-to-date guideline or review is available.

Other methods of developing criteria

Where no criteria are available from clinical guidelines, the following methods may be used for developing criteria based on research evidence.

Prioritising the evidence method

This method of developing criteria reviews the evidence in the source guidelines or systematic reviews for each element of care identified as important in determining outcome (Fraser *et al.*, 1997). The criteria that have most impact on outcome are then categorised as 'must do' or 'should do' (Tables 5 and 6). The process can be summarised as follows.

- Identify key elements of care from review of good-quality guidelines or systematic reviews.
- Carry out focused systematic literature reviews in relation to each key element of care to develop, when it is justified by evidence, one or more criteria for each element of care.
- Prioritise the criteria into 'must do' or 'should do' on the strength of research evidence and impact on outcome.
- Present the criteria in a protocol.
- Include data collection forms, instructions etc.
- Submit the protocol to external peer review.

Table 5. Essential ('must do') criteria for reviewing benzodiazepine prescribing. There is firm research evidence to justify their inclusion (Shaw and Baker, 2001)

- New benzodiazepine prescriptions must only be issued for short-term relief (no longer than four weeks) of severe anxiety or insomnia
- The records show that a patient receiving a prescription (either new or repeat) for a benzodiazepine has been advised on non-drug therapies for anxiety or insomnia
- The records show that the patient has been given appropriate advice on the risks, including the potential for dependence
- The records show that patients prescribed benzodiazepines are reviewed regularly, at least three-monthly

Table 6. Additional ('should do') criteria for benzodiazepine prescribing. There is some research evidence for these criteria, but their impact on outcome is less certain (Shaw and Baker, 2001)

- The records show that, if the patient is aged 65 years or over, they or their carer(s) have been given advice on the risks for elderly patients
- Chronic users (use for 4 weeks or longer) should be identified and encouraged to reduce
- The drug taper should be gradual, with a reduction of 2–2.5 mg diazepam equivalent every 2 weeks
- Before drug reduction is started, the patient has been switched to an equivalent dose of diazepam

RAND/UCLA appropriateness method

This modified panel process, based on the RAND appropriateness method, was originally developed for assessing the performance of various investigative and surgical procedures in the USA (Kahn *et al.*, 1986). The findings of a literature review are submitted to a panel of clinicians, chosen for their clinical expertise and professional influence, who are asked to rate the appropriateness of a set of possible indications for the particular procedure on a 9-point scale from 1 (extremely inappropriate) to 9 (extremely appropriate). A first round of ratings is undertaken without allowing any discussion between the panellists, and a second round is undertaken after a structured panel meeting.

Criteria for assessing the care of people with stable angina, asthma, and non-insulin-dependent diabetes have been developed in the UK using an updated version of these methods (Campbell *et al.*, 1999). Ratings of expert panels can closely reflect the views of clinicians (Ayanian *et al.*, 1998), but different panels produce slightly different criteria, and when they are used to evaluate the quality of care, very different results may be obtained (Shekelle *et al.*, 1998).

The advantages of this method are that it:

- combines systematic review of the scientific literature with expert opinion
- yields specific criteria that can be used for review criteria or practice guidelines, or both
- provides a quantitative description of the expert judgement of a multidisciplinary group of practitioners
- gives equal weight to each panellist in determining the final result.

AHCPR method

Yet another method of developing criteria from guidelines has been produced by the Agency for Health Care Policy and Research (AHCPR), with its own evidence-based guidelines as the starting point (Agenda for Health Care Policy and Research, 1995a and 1995b). The procedure is relatively complex, because the guidelines cover most elements of care, taking note of different levels of evidence. The method uses a panel to rate elements of care on the basis of their importance to quality of care and feasibility for monitoring (Hadorn *et al.*, 1996). Several sets of criteria have been developed in the UK from guidelines supplemented by consultation with expert panels (Hutchinson *et al.*, 2000).

Criteria based on professional consensus

If criteria incorporate or are based on the views of professional groups, it is better to use formal consensus methods. However, different consensus groups are likely to produce different criteria. A checklist is useful to ensure that an explicit process is used to identify, select, and combine the evidence for the criteria, and that the strength of the evidence is assessed in some way (Naylor and Guyatt, 1996).

Several sets of locally based criteria have been developed by involving clinical experts and consensus panels. For example, in an initiative to transfer outpatient follow-up after cardiac surgery from secondary to primary care, protocols for optimal care in general practice were developed in collaboration with a consultant cardiologist, with the criteria and standards being agreed between the cardiologist, general practitioners and nurses (Lyons *et al.*, 1999). Locally developed criteria have the advantage that it is easier to take into account local factors such as the concerns of local users.

In practice, the most efficient approach is likely to be the use of criteria developed by experts from evidence, together with criteria based on the preferences of users determined locally.

Involving users

Practitioners and users may assess the quality of care in different ways. Practitioners are likely to place greater value on clinical competence and measurable benefits to patient health status or outcome. Users, on the other hand, although they value competence, might also be concerned that a holistic approach to care is adopted and be more interested in process criteria. In addition, different patient groups will have different perspectives. For example, older people may have very specific views on communication skills, convenience and accessibility (Table 7). Issues like these need to be translated into measurable criteria in collaboration with healthcare professionals.

Table 7. Outcome measures that older people may consider important (Kelson, 1999)

- The attitude and manner in which a treatment or intervention was carried out
- The effect of treatment and care on quality of life and socio-psychological and emotional outcomes, as well as purely clinical outcomes
- The level and effectiveness of cooperation between different sectors and agencies, taking into account the older person's expectations, aspirations, and preferences

Service users can also become usefully involved in developing criteria that take account of the needs of people with their particular condition, from specific age groups, or ethnic or social backgrounds. Audit teams can collaborate with users to establish their experience of the service and the important elements of care from which criteria can be developed. Several qualitative methods are available to help with understanding users' experiences. These include:

- the critical incident technique (Powell *et al.*, 1994)
- focus groups (Kelson *et al.*, 1998)
- consumer audit (Fitzpatrick and Boulton, 1994).

In a focus group involving people who had suffered strokes and their carers, perceived deficiencies were reported in:

- diagnosis
- treatment and care in hospital

- short-term access to rehabilitation after discharge
- long-term access to rehabilitation services
- access to information and advice on support services at all stages of the recovery process (Kelson *et al.*, 1998).

Once the preferences of users have been identified, they must be incorporated into the criteria. The best way of doing this has not yet been determined, but some basic principles can be followed.

- If the criteria selected by clinicians and those selected by users relate to different elements of care, both sets of criteria may be included.
- If clinicians and users have different views about the same element of care, an open approach is required to achieve consensus.

Additional information may be needed to clarify any differences, which may be less than first thought. Patients or their representatives should then take part in a facilitated discussion with clinicians until agreement can be reached. A situation in which one or other group is made vulnerable or is overruled should be avoided.

Using performance levels

Information about what other teams have achieved can indicate how well a unit is performing in relation to others and encourage the exchange of ideas about how practice can be improved. However, the literature review did not find any evidence that setting a level of performance is more likely to lead to improvements in care after an audit. (Remember that 'performance level' is used in preference to 'standard' in this book.)

Failure to reach a set performance level must be examined carefully, as the reasons may not be obvious. For example, in one audit of treatment for atrial fibrillation, only 50% of eligible patients received warfarin (Howitt and Armstrong, 1999). At first sight, this failed to meet the level of performance suggested by research evidence to be achievable, but further investigation showed that the remaining patients were either too ill, were unable to consent, or could not be persuaded that treatment would benefit them. In other words, the levels of performance achieved in trials are helpful, but should not be regarded as uniformly achievable in unselected patient populations. On the other hand, attempts to exceed the levels suggested by research should not be inhibited.

Benchmarking

Clinical practice benchmarking can be used to set and maintain target levels of performance. An organisation first identifies the areas of practice where the quality of patient care would benefit from comparison and sharing of information about the processes involved in achieving high performance. Then it compares its performance with that of its most successful 'competitors' and considers areas for development in the light of the comparison. An organisation performing less well may seek the advice of one performing well. A process of further comparison and evaluation is required to show development (Ellis, 2000).

The Department of Health publication *The Essence of Care. Patient-Focused Benchmarking for Health Care Practitioners* (Department of Health, 2001) contains benchmarking tools related to eight aspects of care:

- principles of self-care
- food and nutrition
- personal and oral hygiene
- continence and bladder and bowel care
- pressure ulcers
- record keeping
- safety of clients/patients with mental health needs in acute mental health and general hospital settings
- privacy and dignity.

In Wales, *Fundamentals of Care Project* (National Assembly for Wales, 2001), which aims to improve the quality of fundamental aspects of health and social care for people who are acutely or chronically ill, frail or disabled, covers eleven aspects of care for adults:

- dignity
- oral care
- personal care
- sensory care
- pressure area care
- bladder and bowel care
- eating and drinking
- communication
- controlling pain and discomfort
- safety
- promoting independence.

NHS Beacon sites

NHS Beacon sites (www.nhs.uk/beacons) provide a programme of learning opportunities for individuals and teams. At the core of the programme are learning activities – interactive events hosted by Beacons during which small groups of participants share ideas that can be used by other healthcare organisations to benchmark their own services.

In Wales, the National Assembly's Innovations in Care Team (IiC) coordinate the best practice programme, which includes seedcorn funding for innovative schemes, learning events, and information on best practice. The National Assembly for Wales' Clinical Governance Support and Development Unit (CGSDU) provides learning opportunities through clinical governance network support arrangements.

Care pathways

Integrated care pathways define the expected timing and course of events in the care of a patient with a particular condition (Kitchiner and Bundred, 1996). They describe explicitly all the expected processes of care. The topics selected are usually high-volume conditions, and the development of the pathway begins with a review of the scientific evidence. A group consisting of representatives of all the staff involved in care identifies key milestones and maps the process so that duplications or wasteful activities can be highlighted.

A care pathway indicates how care should be provided at each stage of the patient's management and makes measuring performance easier. A copy of the pathway can be included in the patient's records, to be used by all professional groups caring for the patient. This minimises duplication and documentation, and allows variations from the pathway to be identified and investigated, and appropriate action to be taken.

Care pathways are easier to introduce when there is established routine practice and little variation between users. Their introduction requires appreciable time and effort, but they offer an alternative approach that incorporates both systems of care and clinical management. More pathways have been written for the management of surgical than medical conditions. Although detailed evidence about their benefits is limited, encouraging reports from some services are available. For example, the introduction of care pathways over a period of eight years in one hospital was associated with improvements in the management of several conditions (Layton *et al.*, 1998).

References

Agency for Health Care Policy and Research. *Using Clinical Practice Guidelines to Evaluate Quality of Care. Volume 1: Issues. AHCPR publication no 95-0045.* US Department of Health and Human Services, 1995a.

Agency for Health Care Policy and Research. *Using Clinical Practice Guidelines to Evaluate Quality of Care. Volume 2: Methods. AHCPR publication no 95-0046.* US Department of Health and Human Services, 1995b.

Ayanian JZ, Landrum MB, Normand SL, Guadagnoli E, McNeil BJ. Rating appropriateness of coronary angiography – do practising physicians agree with an expert panel and with each other? *New England Journal of Medicine* 1998; **338**: 1896–1904.

Baker R, Fraser RC. Development of audit criteria: linking guidelines and assessment of quality. *British Medical Journal* 1995; **31**: 370–3.

Campbell SM, Roland MO, Shekell PG, Cantrill SA, Buetow SA, Cragg DK. Development of review criteria for assessing the quality of management of non-insulin dependent diabetes mellitus in general practice. *Quality in Health Care 1999*; **8**: 61–5.

Department of Health. *The NHS Plan: A Plan for Investment – A Plan for Reform*. London: The Stationery Office, 2000.

Department of Health. *The Essence of Care. Patient-Focused Benchmarking for Health Care Practitioners*. London: Department of Health, 2001.

Dixon N. *Good Practice in Clinical Audit – A Summary of Selected Literature to Support Criteria for Clinical Audit*. London: National Centre for Clinical Audit, 1996.

Ellis JM. Sharing the evidence: clinical practice benchmarking to improve continuously the quality of care. *Journal of Advanced Nursing* 2000; **32**: 215–25.

Fitzpatrick R, Boulton M. Qualitative methods for assessing health care. *Quality in Health Care* 1994; **3**: 107–13.

Fraser RC, Khunti K, Baker R, Lakhani M. Effective audit in general practice: a method for systematically developing audit protocols containing evidence-based audit criteria. *British Journal of General Practice* 1997; **47**: 743–6.

Hadorn DC, Baker DW, Kamberg CJ, Brook RH. Phase II of the AHCPR-sponsored heart failure guideline: translating practice recommendations into review criteria. *Journal on Quality Improvement* 1996; **22**: 265–76.

Hearnshaw HM, Harker RM, Cheater FM, Baker RH, Grimshaw GM. Expert consensus on the desirable characteristics of review criteria for the improvement of healthcare quality. *Quality in Health Care* 2001; **10**: 173–8.

Howitt A, Armstrong D. Implementing evidence based medicine in general practice: audit and qualitative study of antithrombotic treatment for atrial fibrillation. *British Medical Journal* 1999; **318**: 132–47.

Hutchinson A, McIntosh A, Anderson JP, Gilbert CL, Field R. *Evidence Based Review Criteria for Type 2 Diabetes Foot Care*. Sheffield: RCGP Effective Clinical Practice Unit, University of Sheffield, 2000.

Institute of Medicine. *Guidelines for Clinical Practice: From Development to Use*. Washington DC: National Academic Press, 1992.

Irvine D, Irvine S. *Making Sense of Audit*. Oxford: Radcliffe Medical Press, 1991.

Kahn LK, Roth CP, Fink A, Keesey J, Brook RH, Park RE, Chassin MR, Solomon DH. *Indications for Selected Medical and Surgical Procedures – a Literature and Ratings of Appropriateness*. Colonoscopy. RAND R-3204/5-CWF/HF/PMT/RWJ. Santa Monica, 1986.

Kahn LK, Rubenstein LV, Sherwood MJ, Brook RH. *Structured Implicit Review for Physician Implicit Measurement of Quality of Care: Development of the Form and Guidelines for Its Use*. RAND note N-3016-HCFA. Santa Monica, 1989.

Kelson M. *A Guide to Involving Older People in Local Clinical Audit Activity: National Sentinel Audits Involving Older People*. London: College of Health, 1999.

Kelson M, Ford C, Rigge M. *Stroke Rehabilitation: Patients' and Carers' Views*. London: Royal College of Physicians, 1998.

Kitchiner D, Bundred P. Integrated care pathways. *Archives of Disease in Childhood* 1996; **75**: 1668.

Layton A, Moss F, Morgan G. Mapping out the patient's journey: experiences of developing pathways of care. *Quality in Health Care* 1998; 7 **Suppl**: S30–6.

Lyons C, Thomson A, Emmanuel J, Sharma R, Robertson D. Transferring cardiology out-patient follow-up from secondary to primary care. *Journal of Clinical Governance* 1999; **7**: 52–6.

National Assembly for Wales. *Fundamentals of Care Project*. Cardiff: National Assembly for Wales, 2001.

Naylor CD, Guyatt GH. Users' guide to the medical literature IX. How to use an article about a clinical utilization review. *Journal of the American Medical Association* 1996; **275**: 1435–9.

Powell J, Lovelock R, Bray J, Philp I. Involving users in assessing service quality: benefits of using a qualitative approach. *Quality in Health Care* 1994; **3**: 199–202.

Royal College of Nursing. *Quality Patient Care – the Dynamic Standard Setting System*. Harrow: Scutari, 1990.

Scottish Intercollegiate Guidelines Network. *Secondary Prevention of Coronary Heart Disease Following Myocardial Infarction*. Edinburgh: Scottish Intercollegiate Guidelines Network, 2000 (www.sign.ac.uk).

Shaw E, Baker R. Audit protocol: benzodiazepine prescribing in primary care. *Journal of Clinical Governance* 2001; **9**: 45–50.

Shekelle PG, Kahan JP, Bernstein SJ, Leape LL, Kamberg CJ, Park RE. The reproducibility of a method to identify the overuse and underuse of medical procedures. *New England Journal of Medicine* 1998; **338**: 1888–95.

Stage Three: measuring level of performance

Key points

- Patient registers are used to identify patients, but registers can be incomplete. The identification of patients using several sources can be an appropriate response.
- Although clinical records are frequently used as the source of data, they are often incomplete. The collection of data from several sources can help to overcome this problem.
- When collecting data, a carefully developed data abstraction tool is recommended. Training data abstractors can improve data consistency.
- If routinely collected data are available, they may be appropriate for use in audit.
- Electronic information systems can contribute to audit in many ways, including: improving access to research evidence; identifying users; collecting data; prompting change through record templates; and enabling revised systems of care to be introduced.

Key notes

- Health service professionals must be aware of the ethical implications of audit and their responsibilities under the Data Protection Act (1998) when collecting data and presenting results.
- Every audit should define the users to be included, the aspects of care under review, and the time period over which the criteria apply.
- Health service professionals need to be able to apply appropriate sampling techniques.

Planning data collection

To make sure that the data collected are precise, and that only essential data are collected, certain details about what is to be audited must be established from the outset. These are:

- the user group to be included, with any exceptions noted (Table 8)
- the healthcare professionals involved in the users' care
- the time period over which the criteria apply.

Table 8. Examples of statements (or 'inclusion criteria') that define specific populations for the purposes of particular audits

- All children under 16 years diagnosed with asthma and registered with the primary healthcare team
- All people with multiple sclerosis in a Health Authority area
- All women receiving treatment for breast cancer in England and Wales

Agreement on these points helps to limit the amount of data that have to be collected. It is also important to decide on the type of data analysis that is to be used before data collection starts (*see* page 41).

Staff who are involved in the care process that is to be audited will know the range and reliability of information that may be held about users on computer systems or in patient notes, and administrative staff may have access to further management information. Consultation with these groups can help a team think through what data they really need to collect to monitor those processes that directly affect care.

For example, the effectiveness of physical exercise and stretching in ankylosing spondylitis is measured by recording spinal movement in a standardised way. For an audit to assess the completeness of data collection for users attending both physiotherapy and medical clinics, a consensus group of doctors and physiotherapists defined, after discussion, a minimum dataset consisting of three types of data (Table 9). Patient records were then identified from computerised databases, and data were extracted and recorded on a standard form (Lubrano *et al.*, 1998).

Time periods are often specified to enable data collectors to gather a representative number of cases to monitor performance (an example is given in Table 10). The time period chosen depends on:

- the numbers of cases that are treated on a daily basis
- the number needed to make a confident judgement of care provided.

Identifying users

Identifying service users for audit can be a problem. Variability in the uptake and use of patient registers can give rise to misleading comparisons between groups of users.

Table 9. An example of identifying the data to be collected to audit completeness of data on physiotherapy and medical treatment for ankylosing spondylitis (Lubrano *et al.*, 1998)

- **Measures of spinal movement:**
  - height
  - chest expansion
  - cervical rotation
  - tragus or occiput to wall distance
  - modified Schober's flexion and extension
  - side lumbar flexion
  - intermalleolar abduction
  - interfingertip abduction
- **Medical information:**
  - non-steroidal anti-inflammatory drug usage
  - sulfasalazine usage
  - eye disease
  - aortic incompetence
  - renal disease
- **General information:**
  - exercise frequency
  - duration of early morning stiffness

Table 10. Setting time periods in an audit of GP referrals for lumbar spine radiography (Garala *et al.*, 1999)

- An initial 3-month retrospective audit examined:
  - the number of lumbar spine radiographs requested by GPs
  - the percentage of these with a positive result
  - the percentage of people experiencing a change in their clinical management as a result of radiography
- A prospective audit of the same practices for the same time period 1 year later showed:
  - a 61% reduction in requests for lumbar spine radiographs
  - an increase in those with positive results

In addition, medical coding systems can be very unreliable for identifying users, their conditions, and the nature of their care.

Audit staff must be very careful about the accuracy, timeliness and completeness of clinical records. It can help to use certain data collection strategies, including:

- multiple sources of information
- direct observation
- encounter sheets completed at the time by the healthcare professional.

It is always tempting to collect more data than necessary, but only the minimum amount required by the objectives of the audit should be collected. It is better to improve a single aspect of care than to collect data on 20 items and change nothing. There is an inevitable trade-off between data quality and the costs and practicality of collecting data.

Sampling users

Once the group or population of users has been precisely defined by specifying the 'inclusion criteria', it is time to decide on the records from which data will be collected. It may not always be practical or feasible to include each and every user, and in this case, a representative sample is usually chosen from which inferences about the total population can be made. When choosing a sample, two questions need to be answered.

- How many of the users (study population) do I need to select?
- How do I choose a representative sample?

When the sample size has been determined, the sample can be identified. The number needed in the sample is determined by two factors:

- the degree of confidence wanted in the findings
- resource constraints (time, access to data, costs).

Various methods can be used for calculating sample sizes, depending on the type of data. In audit, it is usual to compare the proportion of users whose care is in accordance with the criteria before changes in care with the proportion after the changes. The calculation of sample size for proportions is relatively simple (*see* the example below), but if the data are in a format other than proportions, statistical advice should be sought.

Sampling methods range from very simple to highly sophisticated. Random sampling should be used whenever possible to minimise the risk of bias. This means that each case in the group is allotted a number, and a published random numbers table (e.g. Altman, 1991) is used to identify the case numbers to include. Pocket calculators and computers can also generate random numbers.

Calculating sample sizes for proportions – an example

A primary care team is planning an audit of the care of people with hypertension. They have 300 people being treated for the disorder, but do not have time to review all the records. They select one key criterion – those on treatment should have had their blood pressure checked and the result should have been below 150/90 mmHg on three occasions in the past 12 months – and hope to achieve a performance level of 70%. They are willing to accept 5% inaccuracy due to sampling – in other words, if their findings give a level of 70%, on 95% of occasions the true value would lie between 65% and 75%. They use the public domain software programme Epi Info to calculate the sample size using these parameters, and the sample required is found to be 155. (Epi Info is produced by the Centers for Disease Control and Prevention in the USA, and may be downloaded from www.cdc.gov/epiinfo.)

Interval sampling

Random sampling assumes that the sample can be drawn from a defined population of users or cases. However, users do not form a static population, and the individuals making up the user population (i.e. those attending clinics, practices or who are admitted to hospital) will change during the audit. In these circumstances, the sample is often determined by intervals of time; for example, people admitted to the coronary care unit from January to March inclusive. This is a reasonable approach provided that admission rates and the quality of care are not influenced by major seasonal factors.

Two-stage sampling

Two-stage sampling may improve efficiency (Alemi *et al.*, 1998). A small sample is selected first, and if unequivocal conclusions can be drawn, no more data are collected. If the results are ambiguous a larger sample is selected.

Rapid-cycle sampling

The traditional audit cycle often involves collecting relatively large amounts of data over a long period, with a similar protracted data collection after changes are introduced. Although this approach, if correctly applied, provides good information about performance, it can make the process of change slow. A recently introduced alternative involves the use of small samples, with many repeated data collections to monitor serious fluctuations or changes in care. The cycle is completed quickly, and reliability is improved by the repeated data collections (Alemi *et al.*, 2000; Plsek, 1999).

The Cancer Services Collaborative (CSC) has used rapid cycles of improvement as a key feature of its quality improvement strategy. PDSA cycles (plan, do, study, act) involve testing change ideas on a small scale, usually on a small number of clinicians and small user samples, before introducing the change to other clinics or user groups. Further information on this method can be found in the Service Improvement Guides available from the CSC on the National Patient's Access Team website (http://195.92.252.217/channels/npat/). An evaluation of the method is available from the Health Services Management Centre at the University of Birmingham (www.hsmc3.bham.ac.uk/hsmc/).

Handling data

Data sources

In an ideal world, if an aspect of care is important enough to be audited, all the necessary data items would have been collected routinely and be readily accessible. In reality, data are often held in several databases, on paper or electronically, in different departments, even different organisations, or may not be collected at all. If the required data are not collected routinely, a specific paper or electronic encounter sheet can be devised for healthcare professionals to record additional information during each consultation.

Existing record and information systems may already be adequate for clinical audit purposes, for example, management information systems may already collect the data required for audit. In addition, the Department of Health has developed sets of performance indicators that can be converted into audit criteria for primary and secondary healthcare (NHS Executive, 1999b), and more will be produced in association with the National Service Frameworks.

As information systems in the NHS are improved, a greater range of data will be readily available (NHS Executive, 1998), including electronic patient records, PACT (Prescription Analysis and Cost) data for primary care prescribers, MIQUEST (software that uses health query language to access, aggregate, and analyse data held in general practice computer systems), patient administration systems (PAS), and quality initiatives already under way. The need for information should be considered when services are re-designed or new systems of work are introduced.

An example of incorporating the need for information into the design of a new system is described by Giles *et al.* (1998). A new clinic for people who had had a myocardial infarction was established in Walsall. An important element of the project was the application of IT, the new clinic being served by a purpose-built database from the outset. The database holds the users' clinical records and is used to generate routine correspondence to GPs and users. It also provides a 100% concurrent audit record and a recall mechanism for those overdue for testing. In their paper, the authors conclude that the use of IT had contributed to the success of the project and had improved clinical practice – the proportion of people treated with lipid-lowering drugs increased, and compliance with re-testing was almost complete.

In an audit undertaken in response to concern about the poor referral rate for cardiac rehabilitation, essential referral data were established and an electronic referral pathway through the electronic patient record was developed (Kalayi *et al.*, 1999). An earlier project had determined referral patterns, and these were fed back to the ward managers and cardiologists. Electronic referral took a maximum of 2 minutes compared with approximately 5 minutes for the manual system. The results confirmed that targeted and clinically relevant audit can lead to change, and that IT systems developed to meet clinical needs can provide audit data cost-effectively. IT can also benefit staff and users by saving time in the referral and identification of users.

Individual user

AUDIT PERIOD: 12 MONTHS PRIOR TO DATE OF DATA COLLECTION

Age	
Id No.	

CRITERION 1 History and examination			
(a) Record of:			
Leakage on exertion	y	n	dk
Volume of loss	y	n	dk
Nocturia	y	n	dk
Frequency	y	n	dk
Urgency	y	n	dk
Dysuria	y	n	dk
Dribbling	y	n	dk
(b) Bladder chart	y	n	dk
(c) Record of examination:			
Abdominal	y	n	dk
Pelvic	y	n	dk
Rectal if appropriate	y	n	dk

CRITERION 2 Urinalysis			
Urine dipstick performed	y	n	dk
or			
MSUS sent (symptoms, ± abnormal dipstick)	y	n	dk

CRITERION 3			
PVR volume measured	y	n	dk

CRITERION 4			
Presumed type identified	y	n	dk
If yes:			
Stress	y	n	dk
Mixed	y	n	dk
Overflow	y	n	dk

CRITERION 5 Risk factors assessed and documented			
Medication review	y	n	dk
Atrophic vaginitis	y	n	dk

CRITERION 6 Risk factors assessed/ documented			
BMI	y	n	dk
Constipation	y	n	dk
Smoking	y	n	dk

Figure 4. Audit of the management of urinary incontinence: data collection form for an individual user. From Cheater *et al.*, 1998. (Reproduced with permission from Director, Eli Lilly National Clinical Audit Centre.)

Data abstraction tools

Data for an audit are generally collected retrospectively, in other words some time after care has been provided. Typically, the data are collected from records, and may be extracted onto standard forms or entered directly into a computer database. Figure 4 shows a data collection form used in an audit of the assessment of urinary incontinence by community nurses. Data collection forms must specify precisely the information to be abstracted from the record, and they should be clear and easy to use.

It is good practice to pilot the data collection form to enable any inherent problems to be detected and corrected. Different data collectors will inevitably interpret some record entries in the same record in different ways. It is essential that data collectors undergo training on the use of the data collection form, so any confusing items are identified and a clear policy is established on how data items should be recorded.

A protocol should also be provided for data collectors to follow when deciding whether the patient notes provide sufficient information to suggest that a criterion has definitely been met. Data collectors should be able to seek advice if they encounter entries in records that are particularly confusing. Before starting an audit, the reliability of data collection should be checked by asking data collectors to independently extract data from the same sample of records and then compare their findings. The percentage of items that are the same, or the kappa statistic, is calculated to estimate inter-rater reliability (Altman, 1991). If reliability is low, the data collection procedures must be reviewed.

Retrospective or concurrent data collection?

Retrospective data collection provides a picture of care provided during a time period in the past, for example, the previous six months. Although this provides a baseline of care provision, it may not be as useful as working with concurrent data.

Concurrent data collection gives a team more immediate feedback on its current performance and can act as a positive reinforcement to improve or maintain practice. Concurrent data can be collected and presented on paper or electronically. Appropriately designed and used electronic records can also provide concurrent data that can be used to support the continuous improvement of practice. As IT systems in the NHS improve, concurrent audit and continuous improvement are likely to become more common.

Concurrent data collection and analysis have been used to improve the timeliness of giving thrombolytics to people admitted to an accident and emergency department with chest pain (Plsek, 1999). Each time thrombolytic therapy was administered, a cross was placed in the appropriate 10-minute column of a check-sheet to indicate the time elapsed since presentation. As the histogram eventually developed, the mean, spread, and characteristic shape of the time distribution could be read directly from the check-sheet (Figure 5).

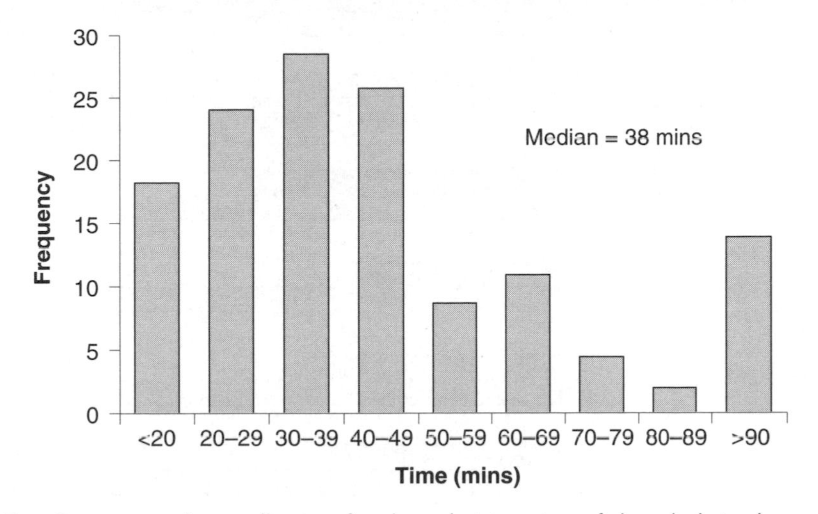

Figure 5. Concurrent data collection for the administration of thrombolytic therapy in the accident and emergency department ('door-to-needle time') (Kendall and McCabe, 1996).

Data analysis

The type of analysis to be used should be identified at an early stage, as it influences both the type and amount of data collected. The analysis can range from a simple calculation of percentages, through to relatively sophisticated statistical techniques. On most occasions, however, simple methods are preferable, and indeed, if the results are to stimulate change, the analysis must be simple enough for everyone in the care process to understand (Plsek, 1999). Furthermore, provided samples have not been used, statistical tests are superfluous. If samples have been taken, the most appropriate calculation to perform is confidence intervals (Gardner and Altman, 1989).

Just as the analysis should be as simple as possible, the findings should be presented simply and clearly. Bar charts have become the most common format, but the numbers should be available in separate tables rather than presenting the charts alone. The example in Figure 6 demonstrates methadone prescribing issues audited in 16 general practices. From these findings, it was possible to draw some conclusions about the impact of the audit and the education sessions on the prescribing practice of the general practitioners involved (Beaumont, 1997).

Statistical quality control charts can help to develop understanding of process performance and provide longitudinal information that may not otherwise be detected. For example, a control chart of the number of patient falls per month, with non-constant control limits due to the varying number of patients, shows three atypical out-of-control events in an otherwise stable process (Figure 7) (Benneyan, 1998).

Although more sophisticated statistical procedures can be used to analyse audit data, expert advice should be sought while the audit is being prepared if this level of analysis is thought to be necessary.

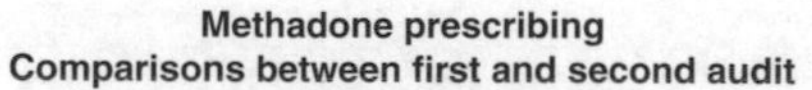

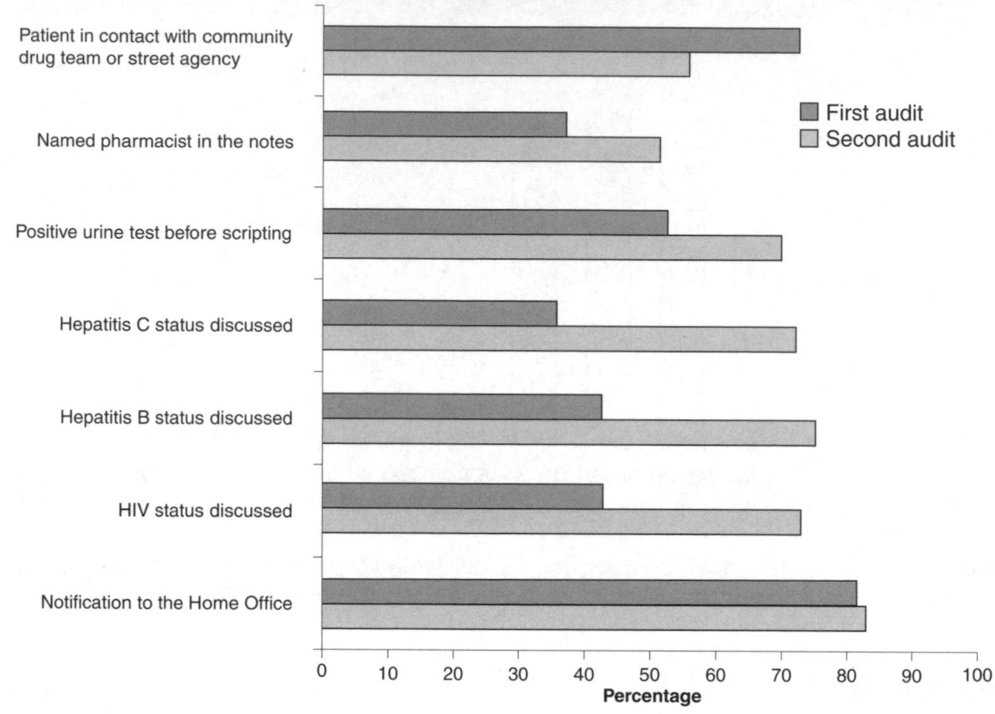

Figure 6. An example of a bar chart used in a clinical audit (data from Beaumont, 1997).

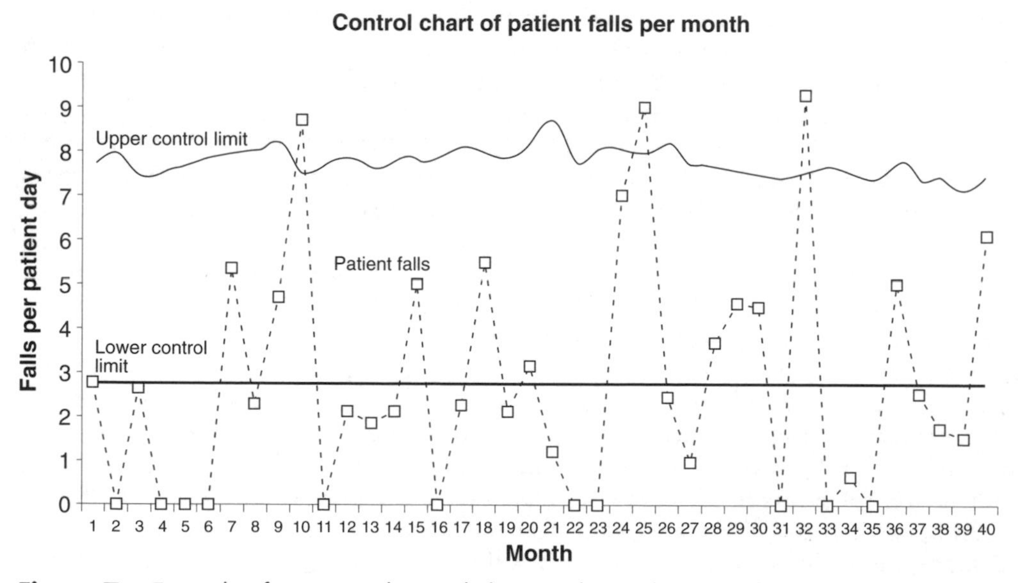

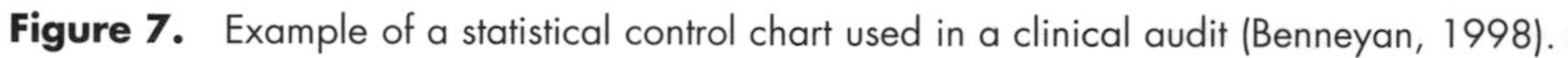

Figure 7. Example of a statistical control chart used in a clinical audit (Benneyan, 1998).

Qualitative analysis

A data collection strategy may include descriptive elements, such as additional comments within a questionnaire or transcripts from focus groups or interviews. These can be analysed qualitatively – qualitative analysis is concerned with words rather than with numbers, and qualitative methods provide a means of assimilating a rich source of information on people's experiences around a clinical topic. Analysis of transcribed tape-recorded interviews or free text comments in questionnaires can be a time-consuming but rewarding exercise, which often produces ideas for improvement in healthcare that can be explored further.

Before the use of qualitative data is considered, the relevant publications should be consulted (Mays and Pope, 2000; Pope *et al.*, 2000) and the help of a skilled analyst enlisted.

Quantitative analysis is concerned with numerical data – the more common form of data in audit. Many of the examples of audit included in this book employ quantitative analysis.

Electronic data capture

Increasing use of computerised patient records means that data collection for clinical audit is becoming easier and more complete, because more data can be automatically transferred to a pre-designed data collection sheet, or analysed directly. In some NHS organisations, electronic records have replaced paper notes. As with any form of data handling, however, planning and consistent recording are needed if the data are to be usable:

- the data to be recorded must be agreed
- professionals must use the system in a consistent manner
- data retrieval must be simple and efficient.

Leadership and organisational commitment to developing an efficient information handling system, as well as suitable software, are needed to make electronic data capture work.

The NHS Information Authority runs several projects relevant to making effective use of computer-held data for clinical audit (Table 11). The Health, Information, Management, Technology and Estates (HIMTE) Division of the National Assembly for Wales is, at the time of press, developing an Information, Management and Technology (IM&T) Plan, which will identify how clinical data systems can become the core of care systems.

The Data Protection Act

Data collection has ethical implications for healthcare staff and users. Several professional bodies have issued written guidance on this issue. The GMC booklet

Table 11. NHS projects to promote effective use of computer-held data. For information on all these resources visit the NHS Information Authority (NHS IA) website at www.nhsia.nhs.uk

- Primary Care Information Services (PRIMIS) – a training and support service to help primary care organisations improve care through the effective use of their computer systems. PRIMIS help primary care staff in the use of MIQUEST software to extract and analyse their own data. Once a practice becomes confident in using the system, MIQUEST can be used to meet clinical governance agendas, National Service Framework implementation etc. (*see* www.exeter.nhsia.nhs.uk/products/vaprod/miquest/miquest.asp and the PRIMIS website (www.primis.nhs.uk)
- Central Cardiac and Audit Database (CCAD) – originally set up in 1996, the CCAD has successfully developed a data collection and analysis service. It is now being used to support targets in the Coronary Heart Disease National Service Framework covering acute myocardial infarction and paediatric cardiac surgery
- Performance Analysis Toolkit – Microsoft Excel-based software package that presents analysis of national inpatient and day-case data to help Health Authorities, primary care organisations, and provider trusts understand and compare the inpatient care received by their local population and the ways in which care is delivered. Includes data about admission rates and provider performance
- Maternity Care Data Project – a project to identify an 'overall pool' of data to be recorded consistently across health organisations by 2003. The data items will support audit and clinical research
- National Clinical Audit Support Programme (NCASP) – to assist clinicians undertaking comparative audit, in recognition of the importance of clinical audit to so many areas within the NHS IA portfolio (including electronic patient record, dataset, and analytical tools development)

Confidentiality: Protecting and Providing Information is a recent example, and those undertaking audit should be familiar with its advice (General Medical Council, 2000).

The GMC suggests the following approach that, if followed, is consistent with the requirements of the Data Protection Act, which came into force on 1 March 2000 (Data Protection Act, 1998).

- When information is gathered directly from patients, auditors must explain why the information is needed and what will happen to it, before asking for the patient's consent.
- If information is obtained from medical records, either patients must consent to identifiable data being used, or a member of the healthcare team should make the information anonymous before it is used in audit.
- If neither of these approaches is possible, it may be permissible for someone from outside the team, who is suitably trained and subject to a duty of confidentiality, to collect the data from the records and make it anonymous without seeking patient consent.

If the last approach is taken, users (patients as referred to by the GMC) should be informed in general terms about how information about them may be used and should be given a chance to object. Before adopting this approach, it is wise to seek the advice of the local district research ethics committee or the GMC.

The UKCC (the Nursing and Midwifery Council from April 2002), offers advice about data confidentiality matters and the latest information on UK and European legislation can be obtained from the Office of the Information Commissioner (www.dataprotection.gov.uk; helpline: 01625 545 745).

These issues of confidentiality and consent are ones that the organisation should address early in order to provide guidance, ideally in the form of a policy to which individuals or teams can refer. NHS organisations should appoint Caldicott guardians who can advise on local arrangements and who are responsible for:

- agreeing and reviewing internal protocols governing the protection and use of user-identifiable information by staff in the organisation
- disclosure of user-identifiable information across organisational boundaries under the auspices of clinical governance (NHS Executive, 1999a; Welsh Office, 1999).

At the time of press, the Office of the Information Commissioner has issued, for consultation, draft guidance on the use and disclosure of medical data; policy and guidance in this area is subject to change (www.doh.gov.uk/ipu).

References

Alemi F, Moore S, Headrick L, Neuhauser D, Hekelman F, Kizys N. Rapid improvement teams. *Joint Commission Journal on Quality Improvement* 1998; **24**: 119–29.

Alemi F, Neuhauser D, Ardito S, Headrick L, Moore S, Hekelman F, Norman L. Continuous self-improvement: systems thinking in a personal context. *Joint Commission Journal on Quality Improvement* 2000; **26**: 74–86.

Altman DG. *Practical Statistics for Medical Research*. London: Chapman and Hall, 1991.

Beaumont B. Methadone prescribing in general practice. *Audit Trends* 1997; **5**: 90–95.

Benneyan JC. Use and interpretation of statistical quality control charts. *International Journal for Quality in Health Care* 1998; **10**: 69–73.

Cheater F, Lakhani M, Cawood C. *Audit Protocol: Assessment of Patients with Urinary Incontinence*. CT14. Leicester: Eli Lilly National Clinical Audit Centre, Department of General Practice & Primary Health Care, University of Leicester, 1998.

Data Protection Act 1998. www.hmso.gov.uk/acts/acts1998/19980029.htm (accessed June 2000).

Garala M, Craig J, Lee J. Reducing the general practitioner referral for lumbar spine X-ray. *Journal of Clinical Governance* 1999; **7**: 186–9.

Gardner MJ, Altman DG. *Statistics with Confidence*. London: BMJ Publishing Group, 1989.

General Medical Council. *Confidentiality: Protecting and Providing Information*. London: General Medical Council, 2000.

Giles PD, Cunnington AR, Payne M, Crothers DC, Walsh MS. Cholesterol reduction for the secondary prevention of coronary heart disease: a successful multidisciplinary approach to implementing evidence-based treatment in a district general hospital. *Journal of Clinical Effectiveness* 1998; **3**: 156–60.

Kalayi C, Rimmier F, Maxwell M. Improving referral for cardiac rehabilitation – an interface audit. *Journal of Clinical Governance* 1999; **7**: 177–80.

Kendall JM, McCabe SE. The use of audit to set up a thrombolysis programme in the accident and emergency department. *Emergency Medicine Journal* 1996; **13**: 49–53.

Lubrano E, Butterworth M, Hesselden A, Wells S, Helliwell P. An audit of anthropometric measurements by medical and physiotherapy staff in patients with ankylosing spondylitis. *Clinical Rehabilitation* 1998; **12**: 216–20.

Mays N, Pope C. Qualitative research in health care. Assessing quality in qualitative research. *British Medical Journal* 2000; **320**: 50–2.

NHS Executive. *Information for Health. An Information Strategy for the Modern NHS 1998–2005*. London: Department of Health, 1998.

NHS Executive. *Clinical Governance. Quality in the New NHS*. London: Department of Health, 1999a.

NHS Executive. *Quality and Performance in the NHS: Clinical Indicators*. London: Department of Health, 1999b.

Plsek PE. Quality improvement methods in clinical medicine. *Pediatrics* 1999; **103**: 203–14.

Pope C, Ziebland S, Mays N. Qualitative research in health care. Analysing qualitative data. *British Medical Journal* 2000; **320**: 114–16.

Welsh Office. Protecting Patient Identifiable Information: Caldicott Guardians in the NHS. WHC(99)92. Cardiff: Welsh Office, 1999.

Stage Four: making improvements

Key points

- A systematic approach to implementation appears to be more effective. Such an approach includes the identification of local barriers to change, the support of teamwork, and the use of a variety of specific methods.
- An investigation of potential barriers to change assists in the development of implementation plans.
- Teams undertaking audit that are appropriately supported and able to use a variety of techniques can identify potential barriers and develop practical implementation plans.
- Contextual factors influence the likelihood of change. These include the significance of change to service users, the effectiveness of teamwork, and the organisational environment.
- Those planning audits should avoid relying on feedback alone as the method of implementing change; although feedback of data alone can occasionally be effective, change is much more likely if it forms part of a more complex set of change processes/interventions.
- The dissemination of educational materials, such as guidelines, has little effect unless accompanied by the use of selected implementation methods.
- Interactive educational interventions including outreach, service user and/or professional reminders (whether manual or computerised), decision support, and system changes can sometimes, but not always, be effective.
- In audit, the use of multifaceted interventions chosen to suit the particular circumstances is more likely to be effective in changing performance than the use of a single intervention alone.

Key note

- Clinical governance programmes offer a structure to support efforts to make improvements, including personal professional development, support of teams, and clear accountability.

Changing behaviours

Theories of how behaviour changes help to explain the influence of the situation in which the change occurs. These theories are encountered in many different fields, such as education and learning, management, economics, sociology, and psychology. No single theory fully explains the process of change in healthcare settings, nor is it possible for any one person to have a detailed knowledge of every theory. However, appreciating the importance of behavioural factors, the nature of the change being implemented, and the context in which people work is helped by being familiar with some of the theories.

The National Co-ordinating Centre for NHS Service Delivery and Organisation (NCCSDO) has summarised the change management literature and described the context of the modern NHS (Iles and Sutherland, 2001): 'The NHS is a large organisation employing people with a wide range of talents, perspectives and passions. It is a complex organisation, with many different cultures and norms, arising from a number of factors including:

- different socialisation processes of the professions
- different needs and expectations of different client groups
- the different histories of different institutions
- local priorities, resource allocation, and performance management.'

Change can occur at organisational, group, or individual levels.

Organisational change

Organisations can be thought of as existing in a state of quasi-equilibrium, in which driving forces are opposed by restraining forces, with the net effect that changes in the organisation are minimised (Table 12) (Rosenfield and Wilson, 1999).

Table 12. Potential driving and restraining forces in a hypothetical hospital trust planning to re-design outpatient services to reduce waiting times

Driving forces	Restraining forces
• Patient pressure	**Individuals**
• National policy	• Fear of increased workload
• Demands from referring general practitioners for improved access	• Concern about staffing and mix
	• Loss of control over work patterns
	Organisations
	• Resistant culture
	• Lack of resources
	• Rigid structure

The status quo must be 'unfrozen' to allow change to occur, followed by 'refreezing' to consolidate the new equilibrium. In order to create the imbalance between the driving and restraining forces that is needed for unfreezing, the restraining forces should be selectively removed or reduced. Merely increasing the driving forces will stimulate an increase in the number or strength of the restraining forces.

Group change

Theories of social influence and conformity can be used to explain change within groups that are smaller than whole organisations. A group exerts pressure on its members to conform, and this pressure can be so powerful that individuals not only comply, but come to believe that the group view is valid and adopt it as their own (Hayes, 1994; Robertson, 1999). However, a minority can influence the group if it has a powerful role and makes its case consistently. The minority may increase its power through seeking allies from inside or outside the group.

Individual change

The trans-theoretical model, which was developed for management of people with addictive behaviours, such as smoking (Robertson, 1999), explains individual behaviour change as a transition through a series of five stages:

- precontemplation – the individual has no intention of changing
- contemplation – change is regarded as a possibility in the near future
- preparation – explicit plans are made
- action – the change occurs
- maintenance – the changed behaviour is consolidated.

Progression through each stage is necessary if a change is to occur. No single strategy can encourage someone to progress from precontemplation to maintenance, and different strategies are required at each stage to help a person move on to the next.

Identifying barriers to change

Theories of behaviour change are helpful, but they must be set in a practical framework of preparing plans to improve care. The concept of barriers to change is a feature of many models that draw on different theories of behaviour change. If the barriers to change are identified beforehand, implementation methods can be tailored to overcome them (Robertson *et al.*, 1996). Obstacles to change can be identified in several ways (Table 13), but generally the simplest and most practical method should be used. If implementation fails at the first attempt, a more detailed investigation of the obstacles may be needed.

Table 13. Some methods of identifying barriers to change

- Interviews of key staff and/or users
- Discussion at a team meeting
- Observation of patterns of work
- Identification of the care pathway
- Facilitated team meetings with the use of brainstorming or fishbone diagrams

One relatively practical framework that incorporates the concept of barriers to change has five principal steps (Grol, 1997).

- The required change is clearly defined, based on evidence, and is presented in a way that staff can easily understand.
- The barriers to change are identified (e.g. using the methods in Table 13), including those relating to professionals and to the healthcare organisation.
- Implementation methods are chosen that are appropriate to the particular circumstances, the change itself, and the obstacles to be overcome. An understanding of selected theories of behaviour change may be used to inform the choice of methods.
- An integrated plan is developed for coordinated delivery and monitoring of the interventions. The plan should describe the sequence in which interventions will be made, the staff and resources required to make them, and the target groups.
- The plan is carried out, and progress is evaluated, with modifications to the plan or additional interventions being used as required.

This model and others like it make clear that implementation of change is a process that must be carefully planned and systematically managed. The particular interventions or implementation methods used form only one aspect of the process of improving care.

Implementing change

A recent review of tools, models and approaches to changing management in the NHS (Iles and Sutherland, 2001) provides a helpful overview of how change can be implemented, addressing issues affecting the management of health services rather than just clinical care, which tends to be the focus of clinical audit.

The effectiveness of the available strategies in various settings and for all clinical activities is considered in detail in the literature review that is presented in the accompanying CD-ROM, and in Appendix XI. It confirms that although many interventions are available for implementing change, no single method is always effective. Indeed, a diagnostic analysis should be undertaken to identify factors that will influence the likelihood of change (Table 13) before selecting the most appropriate strategies for implementing change.

Promoting successful audit

Most health professionals have taken part in audit before, and their experiences support the more formal reviews of implementing change – it is possible to change practice, but it is not a simple process. Although participation levels in audit are generally high, the benefits in terms of improved care have usually been modest (Buttery *et al.*, 1995a; Hearnshaw *et al.*, 1998). It is important to understand the reasons for the limited achievements in order to learn how to make audit more effective in the future.

In a recent review of 93 studies concerned with a wide variety of clinical audits involving different professional groups, the barriers to successful audit included:

- lack of resources
- lack of expertise in project design and analysis
- lack of an overall plan for audit
- poor relationships between professional groups or agencies and within teams
- organisational problems, such as lack of a supportive relationship between clinicians and managers (Johnston *et al.*, 2000).

Hierarchical relationships, lack of commitment from senior doctors and managers, poor organisational links between departments, and lack of time and practical support can also be obstacles to nurses taking part in clinical audit and changing practice (Cheater and Keane, 1998).

Different chief executives in a sample of 29 provider organisations allocated different priorities to developing audit, but most felt that fuller integration with other activities would improve effectiveness (Buttery *et al.*, 1995a). Managerially competent, enthusiastic leaders tended to be most effective, but lack of clarity about aims and an over-concentration on data collection were problems.

Factors that promote the success of clinical audit include:

- sound leadership
- a conducive/supportive organisational environment
- structures and systems to support audit, including mechanisms to make data collection easier
- a well-managed audit programme
- addressing a range of issues important to the trust and individual clinicians
- giving adequate attention to all stages of audit (Buttery *et al.*, 1995b; Rumsey *et al.*, 1996a; Johnston *et al.*, 2000; Rumsey *et al.*, 1996b).

In primary care, second data collections to follow up initial audits are often not completed (Hearnshaw *et al.*, 1998), though better organised practices with adequate resources and a positive attitude to audit may be more successful (Chambers *et al.*, 1996).

Establishing the right environment

The environment in which audit is performed needs the appropriate structures in place and a culture that supports them. And many features of the environment for audit are also important for implementation (Table 14). Indeed, as change is so dependent on behavioural factors, the nature of the environment is even more important for implementation than for other aspects of audit.

Individual environments

Individuals need time to devote to implementing improvements, even if they do not have a role in planning the changes. Giving people an opportunity to think through the implications, and to discuss practical issues with others, can make change less of a challenge. Time alone is not sufficient, however, and systems and support must also be available to help individuals improve their existing skills or develop new ones.

Table 14. Aspects of an environment that promote clinical audit

Individuals	Teams	Organisations
Structure		
Time Personal development plans Access to advice about change management Access to a system for reporting concerns Occupational health service available	Leadership Clear and shared objectives Effective communication Training in improvement methods Opportunities for the team to meet to share ideas and develop plans	Explicit commitment to clinical audit within the organisation Clear system for managing a clinical governance programme Staff with responsibility for audit are fully trained and encouraged to develop new solutions to old problems Good systems for understanding the views of users Good communication with other health and social care agencies
Culture		
Positive attitude to audit and improvement Lack of fear – of change and of confronting less than desired or even poor performance	Open to new ideas Focus on the user's experience Interprofessional respect and cooperation	Users' perspectives genuinely regarded as the focus of quality improvement Open to interest from external agencies in quality of performance, and not afraid of inspection 'No blame' approach to errors Audit given a high priority

Effective personal development linked to regular appraisal of needs must be an integral element of quality improvement and is, increasingly, a professional requirement. The organisation's clinical governance structure should provide support for appraisal through formal and informal meetings or management structures, including an accessible occupational health system. The individual healthcare professional should also be able to report concerns about the quality of care, and be able to suggest new ways of working that lead to improvements.

Individuals are most likely to be committed and involved when they feel safe (McCrea, 1999). An individual who is fearful of review and the consequences that might follow mistakes or poor performance will be reluctant to participate in audit, and there is likely to be covert resistance to change. A culture that stimulates commitment to audit and the feeling of safety cannot be created quickly, or by statements of intent. It is created by actions that generate trust. Even data collections that highlight below-average or poor performance can provide opportunities for building trust.

Team environments

At a very basic level, teams must be able to meet together, to discuss their objectives and share ideas about making changes in their work. Once meetings are established, leadership skills are needed to establish effective communication and ensure that everyone is able to contribute (McCrea, 1999). Several techniques can be used to help teams identify ideas for making change successful, for example:

- brainstorming
- force-field analysis
- collecting ideas on sticky notes (Oakland, 1993).

Successful quality improvement requires teams to build commitment and motivation around key aspects of care. Teams tend to focus on their own internal concerns, and systems are needed to enable them to understand the user's experience, which is of central importance. Information from a user survey or forum can help a team to develop a more complete view of its role and duties, and with effective leadership, generate the motivation for change.

Teams require effective leadership, but people do not automatically have the ability to lead a team (Brearley, 2000). Leadership skills can be developed, however, and access to leadership programmes should be available. Effective leadership establishes respect and understanding between different professional groups, and can help openness about performance to replace defensiveness. Organisations also have an important role to play in this process. Managers also need to be aware that teams can become dysfunctional through poor leadership.

Group and individual factors and leadership interact to determine how successful the implementation of change will be. For example, the success of introducing prophylaxis for deep venous thrombosis by orthopaedic surgeons was limited by scientific and non-scientific factors; these included fear of litigation, ease of administration of medication, marketing by drug companies, adoption of the approach by most peers, and unhappy experiences with individual users (Ferlie *et al.*, 1999). The group was also inward-looking, policy formation relied on loose negotiation, distinct leadership was absent, and managers, users, and nurses were not involved. The reporting to managers of adverse incidents, in particular pulmonary embolism, was undertaken informally, and an attempt to set up an audit of pulmonary embolism failed.

Organisational environments

Clinical governance provides an organisational framework for audit and associated activities (Department of Health, 1998). Clear lines of accountability are expected, and chief executives are accountable on behalf of trust boards for assuring the quality of services. Experience of audit in past years has shown that explicit objectives, clear systems for managing audit, and adequate support in terms of staff and facilities are needed (Buttery *et al.*, 1995a). In addition, effective quality improvement depends on the involvement of users in identifying issues for audit. The clinical governance system should include:

- fully functional procedures for professional development
- appraisals
- effective team management
- adverse incident reporting systems.

If an organisation seeks to improve the quality of care through audit, it should regard the experience of service users as the starting point for change (*see* page 10). The organisation must not fear external review by the health service or the public, and must be able to show by its actions that its statements about openness and freedom from blame are genuine.

External relationships

Users and the public

Communication with the local public must be good, and depends on effective communication systems being in place. New arrangements for user involvement were announced in *The NHS Plan* (Department of Health, 2000), and include the following.

- A Patient Advocacy and Liaison Service and a Patient Forum are to be established in each trust.
- All trusts are to ask users for their views on the services they have received.
- Every local NHS organisation is to publish a patient prospectus setting out the range of services available and the ratings users have given them.

- Local authorities are to be given powers to scrutinise the NHS locally.
- Financial rewards to trusts are to be linked to the results of the annual National Patient Survey.
- User versions of guidelines and other forms of information for users about the care of particular conditions are to be routinely available.

These new systems should both inform and consult users, who need information both about what services and care they can expect in general, and about their own individual care.

In Wales, the new arrangements for user involvement, announced in *Improving Health in Wales* (Minister for Health and Social Services, 2001), include:

- Patient Support Managers, to support patients in their dealings with NHS staff
- Local Health Alliances, set up by local health authorities to engage with the community
- a Health and Social Care Charter to clarify how people can access NHS and social care services and the rights and responsibilities of patients
- annual prospectuses, published by all trusts and Local Health Groups, that set out the services available
- a network of 'expert patients' to support individual patients in the treatment of specific conditions.

The arrangements for involving users and the public, described above, could be operated without a real conviction that users are central to improving the quality of care. Leadership from the top of the organisation is required to show that the design of services around the needs of users is possible, rewarding, and necessary.

Health and social care organisations

Changes that are implemented to improve care may have knock-on effects on other agencies: for example, early discharge schemes may affect both health and local social services. In addition, improvement should not stop at organisational boundaries, but follow users as they make use of different services. This means that both day-to-day operational systems and strategic systems are required to ensure close cooperation between agencies. Agencies may also work together to develop shared objectives for quality improvement. Such an approach is essential in the agreement of health improvement programmes and the implementation of National Service Frameworks.

It is often difficult for organisations, teams, and individual professionals to appreciate the consequences of their decisions for other agencies, or to fully understand their working practices. As a result, the other agencies are often misunderstood and a cycle of poor cooperation and recrimination is established. The beliefs and assumptions that are associated with these problems should be challenged. Opportunities to make progress may arise during the course of local audit projects or in the development of policies related to the health improvement programme or National Service Frameworks. Once the user's experience is understood, the importance of improving care across boundaries becomes clear.

Examples of implementing change

The three examples described below share common features and illustrate some of the points discussed in the previous sections. In each case, the changes were developed from evidence about appropriate care and were accepted by the professionals involved. Users were also involved in each example, either in giving their views about aspects of care or the design of services, or by being given additional information based on research evidence to enable them to make an informed decision about their care. The examples also show how multiple interventions were used to improve care. In each case the selection of interventions was based on an appreciation of the local circumstances and the particular obstacles or issues that needed addressing. The planning and coordination involved in each example indicates that in each case the environment was conducive to successful audit.

Antibiotic prescribing for otitis media in children (Cates, 2000)

A Cochrane review questioned the use of antibiotics in the initial management of acute otitis media in children. The doctors in the practice agreed a new policy, but recognised that it might be difficult to implement change. They therefore agreed to offer parents a deferred prescription so that they could wait and see if their child improved without antibiotics. They also prepared an information leaflet for parents explaining the results of research and recommending alternative management, including paracetamol. In the months that followed, fewer children with otitis media were given antibiotics.

Pain control after Caesarean section (Antrobus, 1999)

Pain control was identified as a problem from an audit involving case-note review and interviews with women after Caesarean section. A new protocol was developed from a review of the evidence, and this was supported by formal pain assessments, pre-printed prescription labels to apply to drug charts, and the introduction of self-medication by women. Education was delivered to doctors and nurses in individual face-to-face sessions (as in educational outreach). At the second data collection a few months later:

- women were more satisfied with pain control
- the incidence of pain was reduced
- mobility was improved
- the length of hospital stay was reduced.

Management of acute stroke (Dunning et al., 1999)

An initial audit demonstrated a lack of systematic coordination of care and variability in clinical practice. A project team was established, and an integrated care pathway developed. The communication strategy involved presentations and discussions with members of the directorate, the trust board, and the public, and local councillors. A user support group was set up. New documentation was introduced, and a new psychological assessment framework was adopted. Stroke beds were designated, and the referral process was streamlined.

Subsequent data collections showed that:

- the proportion of people discharged to their own homes had increased
- hospital stays were shorter
- there was a lower incidence of hospital-acquired complications.

References

Antrobus H. Do-it-yourself pain control. *ImpAct* 1999; **1**: 6–7.

Brearley M. Teams: lessons from the world of sport. *British Medical Journal* 2000; **321**: 1141–3.

Buttery Y, Walshe K, Rumsey M, Amess M, Bennett J, Coles J. *Provider Audit in England*. London: CASPE Research, 1995a.

Buttery Y, Rumsey M, Bennett J, Coles J. *Dorset HealthCare NHS Trust's Clinical Audit Programme. A Case Study*. London: CASPE Research, 1995b.

Cates C. Promoting interest in evidence-based practice in primary care. *ImpAct* 2000; **2**: 1–3.

Chambers R, Bowyer I, Campbell I. Investigation into the attitude of general practitioners in Staffordshire to medical audit. *Quality in Health Care* 1996; **5**: 13–19.

Cheater FM, Keane M. Nurses' participation in audit: a regional study. *Quality in Health Care* 1998; **7**: 27–36.

Department of Health. *A First Class Service. Quality in the New NHS*. London: Department of Health, 1998.

Department of Health. *The NHS Plan: A Plan for Investment – A Plan for Reform*. London: The Stationery Office, 2000.

Dunning M, Abi-Aad G, Gilbert D, Hutton H, Brown C. *Experience, Evidence and Everyday Practice. Creating Systems for Delivering Health Care*. London: King's Fund, 1999.

Ferlie E, Wood M, Fitzgerald L. Some limits to evidence-based medicine: a case study from elective orthopaedics. *Quality in Health Care* 1999; **8**: 99–107.

Grol R. Beliefs and evidence in changing clinical practice. *British Medical Journal* 1997; **315**: 418–21.

Hayes N. *Foundations of Psychology*. London: Routledge, 1994.

Hearnshaw H, Baker R, Cooper A. A survey of audit activity in general practice. *British Journal of General Practice* 1998; **48**: 979–81.

Iles V, Sutherland K. *Managing Change in the NHS. Organisational Change. A Review for Health Care Managers, Professionals and Researchers*. London: National Co-ordinating Centre for NHS Service Delivery and Organisation, 2001.

Johnston G, Crombie IK, Davies HTO, Alder EM, Millard A. Reviewing audit: barriers and facilitating factors for effective clinical audit. *Quality in Health Care* 2000; **9**: 23–36.

McCrea C. Good clinical audit requires teamwork. In: Baker R, Hearnshaw H, Robertson N, eds. *Implementing Change with Clinical Audit*. Chichester: Wiley, 1999: 119–32.

Minister for Health and Social Services. *Improving Health in Wales – A Plan for the NHS and its Partners*. Cardiff: National Assembly for Wales, 2001.

Oakland JS. *Total Quality Management. The Route to Improving Performance*. 2nd edition. Oxford: Butterworth-Heinemann, 1993.

Robertson N. A systematic approach to managing change. In: Baker R, Hearnshaw H, Robertson N, eds. *Implementing Change with Clinical Audit*. Chichester: Wiley, 1999: 37–56.

Robertson N, Baker R, Hearnshaw H. Changing the clinical behaviour of doctors – a psychological framework. *Quality in Health Care* 1996; **5**: 51–4.

Rosenfield RH, Wilson DC. *Change in Organizations. Managing Organizations. Text, Readings and Cases*. 2nd edition. Maidenhead: McGraw-Hill, 1999: 283–98.

Rumsey M, Buttery Y, Bennett J, Coles J. *Wythenshawe Hospital's Clinical Audit Programme. A Case Study*. London: CASPE Research, 1996a.

Rumsey M, Buttery Y, Bennett J, Coles J. *North Staffordshire's Joint Clinical Audit Programme. A Case Study*. London: CASPE Research, 1996b.

Stage Five: sustaining improvement

Key points

- Organisations can use recognised assessment techniques to evaluate the quality of audit carried out by healthcare professionals.
- Alternative models of assessing healthcare provision, such as delay pattern analysis and critical incident review, can assist with identifying and investigating certain deficiencies in care. The most effective approaches for ensuring that these methods lead to improved care are uncertain.

Key notes

- Improvements in care implemented as a part of clinical audit must be monitored, evaluated, sustained, and reinforced within a supportive environment.
- Structures and systems must be developed to enable organisations to integrate improvements within a planned strategy.
- A culture is required that makes the user's experience the primary motivation for improvements, creates confident staff who do not fear reporting or confronting inadequate performance, and has clear and constant objectives.
- Systems, structures, and specific mechanisms are available for monitoring sustained improvement.

Although improving performance is the primary goal of audit, sustaining that improvement is also essential. Indeed, any systematic approach to changing professional practice should include plans to:

- monitor and evaluate the change
- maintain and reinforce the change (NHS Centre for Review and Dissemination, 1999).

Monitoring and evaluating changes

Collecting data for a second time, after changes have been introduced, is central to both assessing and maintaining the improvements made during clinical audit. The same procedures of sample selection, information collection, and analysis (*see* Stage Three: measuring level of performance) should be used throughout the process, to ensure that the data are valid and comparable with each other. Rapid-cycle data collection may also be appropriate, in which only absolutely essential data are collected from small samples (again, *see* Stage Three).

If performance targets have not been reached during implementation, modifications to the plan or additional interventions will be needed.

Using IT

A well thought out and integrated IT strategy can help data collection. For example, it is already possible to link a patient record to a specially constructed, audit-collection computer program to record levels of care automatically and continuously. Those with access to the program – individuals, team leaders, and managers with responsibility for quality control – have immediate access to current levels of care (*see* the NHS Beacons Learning Network website, www.nhs.uk/beacons).

It may be easier to sustain improvement within an environment that accepts re-audit at regular intervals. In some cases, regular re-audit is similar to quality control, in which the process continues provided that a sample of events is within the acceptable limits. Again, computerised patient records can provide automatic and instantaneous audit data (www.nhs.uk/beacons; NHS Executive, 1998).

Clinical performance indicators

Time and planning are both needed in setting up systems for long-term monitoring of indicators, and unrealistically short timescales should be avoided. However, although organisations must invest in facilities, personnel, and training to monitor indicators, it is important to realise that only the minimum number of essential indicators should be included in monitoring.

The work involved in third or later data collections can be minimised if monitoring is based on routinely available or easily collected indicators, such as those that contribute to the NHS Performance Assessment Framework (NHS Executive, 1999) and the National Survey of Patient and User Experience (*see* www.doh.gov.uk/nhsperformanceindicators) in England and the Performance Management Framework in Wales.

The small number of high-level, clinical performance indicators being developed for use in the NHS Performance Assessment Framework (England) and the Performance Management Framework (Wales) relate to only a very limited range of care, and they are unlikely to be directly useful on most occasions. However, performance indicators (England) and clinical indicators (Wales) are also being developed within each NHS National Service Framework. For example, the Framework for Coronary Heart Disease (Department of Health, 2000a) includes clinical indicators (Table 15). These indicators draw on existing sources of information whenever possible, to minimise the problem of collecting additional data. If no data source is available and the performance indicator is a key measure, systems for providing data must be created. For example, many primary care organisations do not routinely monitor the proportion of people with recognised coronary heart disease who have been advised about aspirin, and so they will have to develop a monitoring system for this indicator.

Whenever possible, authoritative, evidence-based sources of guidance on selecting performance indicators and advice on audit criteria (such as those in the technology appraisals and guidelines produced by NICE) should be used. Such sources are likely to also be used by other healthcare organisations, which will facilitate comparison of performance. Development of local indicators is sometimes required, but care should be taken to ensure that they are valid and reliable (Sheldon, 1998).

When performance indicators are used to monitor sustained improvement, it is vitally important to ensure that data are collected accurately and analysed and interpreted appropriately. The findings should be reviewed on a regular basis and used

Table 15. Coronary heart disease performance indicators (Department of Health, 2000a)

	Acute myocardial infarction (AMI)	Preventing coronary heart disease among those at high risk
Health improvement	Coronary heart disease mortality rates by Health Authority (from existing public health common dataset)	
Fair access, effective delivery	Number and percentage of patients eligible for thrombolysis receiving it within 60 minutes of call for professional help ('call-to-needle-time')	Number and proportion of people aged 35–74 years with recognised coronary heart disease whose records document advice about the use of aspirin
Efficiency	Reference costs for AMI (HRG codes E11 and E12)	
User experience	National coronary heart disease survey of NHS patients	
Health outcome	Proportion of people aged 35–74 years in a primary care organisation and health authority area with a diagnosis of AMI who die in hospital within 30 days of their infarct	Rate of cardiovascular events in people with a prior diagnosis of coronary heart disease, peripheral vascular disease, transient ischaemic attack, or occlusive stroke

to guide service development. Any decline in performance should be investigated through more detailed audits, and new improvement strategies activated as necessary. In this way, monitoring can be linked to an overall quality strategy and becomes a routine part of managing the service.

Other methods of continued monitoring

Errors, adverse incidents, and significant event audit can also be used for continued monitoring. Comments from users may be included as sources of information about performance. Although these informal mechanisms can detect declining performance and initiate formal investigations, they depend on an environment that fosters the reporting of errors and adverse incidents and they are no substitute for systematic monitoring.

Evaluating audit quality

The quality of clinical audit programmes must be evaluated as part of the wider clinical governance agenda. A useful framework for trusts assessing, reviewing, and improving the effectiveness of their clinical audit programmes has been developed and can be downloaded from www.hsmc3.bham.ac.uk/hsmc (Walshe and Spurgeon, 1997), and a scale to measure the quality of audit projects through audit project reports has been developed and tested (Millard, 2000). CHI undertakes regular reviews of clinical governance in NHS trusts and primary care organisations, and assessment of audit is an integral part of these assessments. The framework currently used by CHI is given in Appendix VII.

A set of checklists is included in this book (Appendix VI), based on the key points and key notes highlighted in each section. The checklists can be used by audit leaders and clinicians to evaluate the methods they have used, or are planning to use, in their audits. They may also help those responsible for managing audit programmes. The checklists are intended as practical aids to learning, and are not designed for external assessments of audits or audit programmes.

Maintaining and reinforcing improvement

Maintaining and reinforcing improvement over time is a complex process. In UK projects in which improvements have been sustained, some common factors have been identified (Dunning *et al.*, 1999), including:

- reinforcing or motivating factors built in by the management to support the continual cycle of quality improvement
- integration of audit into the organisation's wider quality improvement systems
- strong leadership.

In quality improvement initiatives in US hospitals, four interdependent processes have been found to support the lasting impact of clinical audit:

- a strategy that recognises audit activity, combined with an achievable plan of quality improvement
- a culture that supports the concept of planned audit activity, leading to improvements in quality of which everyone in the organisation is aware and supportive
- IT processes that can provide accurate information about the organisation, allowing sensible decisions to be made about where audit is needed and whether changes have had the desired effects
- appropriate structures to support and implement the changes that are suggested (Shortell, 1998).

Appropriate organisational development

Developing and encouraging sustained quality performance by healthcare organisations involves attention to three specific areas of organisational development (Davies and Nutley, 2000; Greenhalgh, 2000; Huntington *et al.*, 2000):

- cultural change, ensuring that the shared values and beliefs of the organisation support the ideas of quality improvement
- adequate training, so that staff can gather and analyse data accurately
- an organisational structure that coordinates and monitors quality improvement work quickly and effectively.

A review of organisational change for quality improvement in healthcare has produced three principal recommendations, which can be described as **vision**, **constancy** and **management** (Garside, 1998).

- The desired end-state or vision should be explicitly articulated, alliances with external organisations should be forged while achieving it, and it should be retained in difficult times of resistance to change.
- Leaders must constantly show commitment to the desired direction of change, and that they mean what they say.
- The details must be managed carefully, for example, by appointing a person to oversee the task, creating project teams, making time available, and arranging for a source of transitional funding to be available.

Using existing frameworks

An organisation may benefit from fitting the planning and reporting of audit into an established framework that already operates at strategic, organisational, and clinical levels (Table 16). At the strategic level, programmes of audit linked to national issues

Table 16. The European Foundation for Quality Management (EFQM) Excellence Model: a strategic quality improvement model. More information on the model and its effectiveness can be found at www.efqm.org

- Concentrates on the whole of an organisation's activities
- Is concerned with internal processes and use of resources as well as performance and outputs
- Applies assessment processes to indicate where an organisation is performing well and where poorly
- Provides clearly defined standards as a baseline for continuous improvement
- Provides results on the basis of which the most effective approaches can be designed and resources deployed
- Provides means of assessing and reviewing the effectiveness of the approaches chosen

are agreed and timetables set out, linked to other aspects of the organisation's development plan. The responsibility for providing education, training, and support for audit teams lies at the organisational level (*see* Stage One: preparing for audit).

Leadership

Leadership plays a vital role in any process of quality improvement. Leadership is not just telling people what to do, but also ensuring that the right resources are being used in the most appropriate way. The pragmatic approach argues that leaders need to create the vision that quality matters and quality issues are worth striving for (Bate, 1998). In essence this means that concern for quality should infuse all aspects of the organisation's work and be sustained through monitoring and re-audit (Berwick, 1996).

Changing the organisational culture

The first three recommendations of the Bristol Royal Infirmary Inquiry (2001) are:

- in a patient-centred healthcare service, patients must be involved, wherever possible, in decisions about treatment and care
- the education and training of all healthcare professionals should be imbued with the idea of partnership between the healthcare professional and the patient
- the notion of partnership between the healthcare professional and the patient, whereby the patient and the professional meet as equals with different expertise, must be adopted by healthcare professionals in all parts of the NHS, including healthcare professionals in hospitals.

These recommendations have been accepted by the Government. The Inquiry Report also says that: 'The culture of the future must be a culture of safety and of quality; a culture of openness and of accountability; a culture of public service; a culture in which collaborative teamwork is prized; and a culture of flexibility in which innovation can flourish in response to patients' needs.' Throughout this book we have sought to make clear the fundamental importance of involving people who use the health service in clinical audit and other methods of quality improvement, and the report of the Bristol Royal Infirmary Inquiry explains why.

Changing the organisational culture is a core aspect of plans to identify and reduce the number of severe adverse incidents in the NHS (Department of Health, 2000b). The ideal culture is informed by four principal elements.

- Staff are prepared to report errors or near-misses, which the organisation analyses and provides feedback on any action being taken.
- The culture is just, and staff are able to trust the organisation to distinguish acceptable from unacceptable behaviours.
- The culture is flexible, respecting the skills and abilities of front-line staff and allowing them to take control.
- The culture is prepared to learn and has the will to implement necessary major reforms.

The learning organisation

An organisation that is committed to quality improvement can be thought of as a learning organisation (Argyris, 1991). This concept distinguishes organisations by how supportive they are to new ideas. A learning organisation is responsive to change and seeks to improve the quality of its output through single-, double- or triple-loop learning.

- Single-loop learning involves incremental change to close the gap between current and target levels of performance.
- Double-loop learning allows organisations to change the existing assumptions about performance, including the goals of the organisation and the levels of performance that can be attained.
- Triple-loop learning generalises developments learnt from one audit to other areas of healthcare, so that improvements are generated simultaneously.

Organisational learning and other aspects of organisational change are discussed in more detail in a guide published by the NHS Service Delivery and Organisation Research and Development Programme (Iles and Sutherland, 2001).

Knowledge management

Knowledge management, another developing area of interest, concentrates on how organisations become more intelligent and work better and more intelligently. This approach (*see* www.eknowledgecenter.com/articles/1010/1010.htm) demonstrates a very important principle: that tacit knowledge of how to improve performance is often already present in an organisation, but is not necessarily shared by the workforce.

Knowledge management recognises that organisations need to develop a culture and structures to spread that knowledge so that it is useful to the organisation.

Sustained quality improvement in practice

Many attempts to support quality improvement by clinical audit have been reported in *NHS Beacons* (NHS Beacon Services, 2000/2001), *ImpAct* (a supplement of *Bandolier, see* Table 17), an Internet site devoted to supporting quality improvement audit projects and quality improvement programmes. Although these examples provide useful reports of the success of quality improvement initiatives, it is not clear how generally applicable they are, because the supporting environments of the projects are often unknown.

Table 17. Quality improvement activities featured in *ImpAct*

Salford – Diabetes Clinical Team
- www.jr2.ox.ac.uk/bandolier/ImpAct/imp04/i4-04.html

South Tees – colposcopy service
- www.jr2.ox.ac.uk/bandolier/ImpAct/imp04/i4-04.html

Leicester – Royal Infirmary Gynaecology Department
- www.jr2.ox.ac.uk/bandolier/ImpAct/imp05/i5-1.html

East Kent – Primary Care Clinical Effectiveness (PRICCE) programme
- www.jr2.ox.ac.uk/bandolier/ImpAct/imp01/EASTKENT.html

Dorset – Successful Cardiac Care based on Evidence of Effectiveness in Dorset (SUCCEED) project
- www.jr2.ox.ac.uk/bandolier/ImpAct/imp09/i9-4.html

CHI, the Modernisation Agency in England and the Innovations in Care (IiC) Team and Clinical Governance Support and Development Unit (CGSDU) at the National Assembly for Wales also have roles in helping to sustain quality improvements in NHS organisations. CHI does this by providing feedback on the implementation of clinical management strategies within organisations in which a wide range of indicators of performance are considered, and the Modernisation Agency (England) and CGSDU (Wales) by facilitating the development of an environment within the NHS in which clinical audit can thrive. Health Authorities are already responding to their responsibilities and creating structures to deal with critical incident reporting and systems for dealing with poorly performing practitioners.

References

Argyris C. Teaching smart people how to learn. *Harvard Business Review* 1991; **69**: 99–109.

Bate SP. *Strategies for Cultural Change*. Oxford: Butterworth-Heinemann, 1998.

Berwick DM. A primer on leading the improvement of systems. *British Medical Journal* 1996; **312**: 619–22.

Davies HTO, Nutley ST. Organisational culture and the quality of the service provided. *Quality in Health Care* 2000; **9**: 111–19.

Department of Health. *National Service Framework for Coronary Heart Disease*. London: Department of Health, 2000a.

Department of Health. *An Organisation with a Memory. Report of an Expert Group on Learning From Adverse Events in the NHS*. London: Department of Health, 2000b.

Dunning M, Abi-Aad G, Gilbert D, Hutton H, Brown C. *Experience, Evidence and Everyday Practice. Creating Systems for Delivering Health Care*. London: King's Fund, 1999.

Garside P. Organisational context for quality: lessons from the fields of organisational development and change management. *Quality in Health Care* 1998; 7 **Suppl**: S8–15.

Greenhalgh T. Change and the organisation: culture and context. *British Journal of General Practice* 2000; **50**: 340–1.

Huntington J, Gillam S, Rosen R. Clinical governance in primary care: organisational development for clinical governance. *British Medical Journal* 2000; **321**: 679–82.

Millard AD. Measuring the quality of clinical audit projects. *Journal of Evaluation of Clinical Practice* 2000; **6**: 359–70.

Iles V, Sutherland K. *Organisational Change. Managing Change in the NHS*. London: National Co-ordinating Centre for NHS Service Delivery and Organisation Research and Development Programme, 2001. (Can be downloaded from www.sdo.lshtm.ac.uk)

NHS Beacon Services. *NHS Beacons Learning Book*, 2000/2001. Petersfield: NHS Beacon Programme (www.nhs.uk/beacons).

NHS Centre for Review and Dissemination. Getting evidence into practice. *Effective Health Care*; **5**. York: University of York, 1999.

NHS Executive. *Information for Health. An Information Strategy for the Modern NHS 1998–2005*. London: Department of Health, 1998.

NHS Executive. *Quality and Performance in the NHS: Clinical Indicators*. London: Department of Health, 1999.

Sheldon T. Promoting health care quality: what role performance indicators? *Quality in Health Care* 1998; 7 **Suppl**: S45–50.

Shortell SM, Bennett CL, Byck GR. Assessing the impact of continuous quality improvement on clinical practice: what it will take to accelerate progress. *Millbank Quarterly* 1998; **76**: 593–624.

Walshe K, Spurgeon P. *Clinical Audit Assessment Framework, HSMC Handbook Series 24*. Birmingham: University of Birmingham, 1997.

Appendix I: glossary

Term	Meaning	Source
Adverse event	An untoward or undesirable occurrence in the healthcare process which has or potentially has some negative impact on a patient or patients and results or may result from some part of the healthcare process	Walshe K. Adverse events in health care: issues in measurement. *Quality in Health Care* 2000; **9**: 47–52.
Benchmarking	A process defining a 'level of care set as a goal to be attained'.	Agency for Health Care Policy and Research. *Using Clinical Practice Guidelines to Evaluate Quality of Care. Volume 2. Methods*. 1995.
Clinical audit	Clinical audit is a quality improvement process that seeks to improve patient care and outcomes through systematic review of care against explicit criteria and the implementation of change. Aspects of the structure, processes, and outcomes of care are selected and systematically evaluated against explicit criteria. Where indicated, changes are implemented at an individual, team, or service level, and further monitoring is used to confirm improvement in healthcare delivery.	This book – *see* page 1.

Clinical effectiveness	The extent to which specific clinical interventions, when deployed in the field for a particular patient or population, do what they are supposed to do, i.e., maintain and improve health and secure the greatest possible health gain from available resources.	NHS Executive. *Promoting Clinical Effectiveness. A Framework for Action In and Through the NHS.* Leeds, 1996.
Clinical governance	... a framework through which the NHS organisations are accountable for continuously improving the quality of their services and safeguarding high standards of care by creating an environment in which excellence in clinical care will flourish.	Department of Health. *A First Class Service: Quality in the New NHS.* HMSO, London, 1998. Welsh Office. *Quality Care and Clinical Excellence.* Cardiff: Welsh Office, 1998.
Clinical guidelines	... systematically developed statements to assist practitioner and patient decisions about appropriate healthcare for specific circumstances	Institute of Medicine. *Guidelines for Clinical Practice: from Development to Use.* Washington, DC: National Academic Press, 1992.
Criteria	Systematically developed statements that can be used to assess the appropriateness of specific healthcare decisions, services, and outcomes.	Institute of Medicine. *Guidelines for Clinical Practice: from Development to Use.* Washington, DC: National Academic Press, 1992.
Evidence-based practice	The conscientious, explicit, and judicious use of current best evidence, based on systematic review of all available evidence – including patient-reported, clinician-observed and research-derived evidence – in making and carrying out decisions about the care of individual patients. The best available evidence, moderated by the patient circumstances and preferences, is applied to improve the quality of clinical judgements.	National Centre for Clinical Audit. *Glossary of Terms Used in the NCCA Criteria for Clinical Audit.* London: National Centre for Clinical Audit, 1997.

Facilitator	In the context of clinical audit, the role of the facilitator is to help the clinical audit group to assimilate the evidence and come to a common understanding of clinical audit methodology, to guide the clinical audit project from planning to reporting and to enable the group to work effectively to that end.	Morrell C, Harvey G. *The Clinical Audit Handbook*. London: Baillière Tindall, 1999.
Health technology appraisals	Technology appraisals provide patients, health professionals, and health service managers with a single, authoritative source of advice on new and existing health technologies.	National Institute for Clinical Excellence website (www.nice.org.uk) Accessed October 2000.
Level of performance	In this book the term 'level of performance' is used in preference to the potentially confusing term 'standard' (*see* page 28).	
National Service Frameworks	National Service Frameworks set national standards and define service models for a specific service or care group, put in place programmes to support implementation, and establish performance measures against which progress within an agreed timescale will be measured.	National Service Frameworks website (www.doh.gov.uk/nsf/nsfhome.htm). Accessed October 2000.
Outcome	Result of an intervention. Outcomes can be desirable, such as improvement in the patient's condition or quality of life, or undesirable, like side-effects.	NHS Executive. *Evidence-Based Health Care. An Open Learning Resource for Health Care Practitioners*. CASP and HCLU, 1999.
Research	A systematic investigation undertaken to discover facts or relationships and reach conclusions using specifically sound methods.	Hockey L. The nature and purpose of research. In: *The Research Process in Nursing*. 3rd edition. London: Blackwell, 1996.
Standard	*See* Stage Two: selecting criteria, page 22.	

Systematic review	A review in which all the trials on a topic have been systematically identified, appraised, and summarised according to predetermined criteria. It can, but need not, involve meta-analysis as a statistical method of adding together the results of trials that meet minimum quality criteria.	*Clinical Evidence*. BMJ Publishing Group and the American College of Physicians, American Society of Internal Medicine, 1999.
User	In this book, the terms 'user' and 'service user' include patients, service users, and carers, and members of groups and organisations that represent their interests.	

Appendix II: online resources for clinical audit

When *Evidence on Good Practice in Clinical Audit* was published in 1996, there was no mention of the world-wide web in the text, or even a single URL listed in the references. One measure of the distance travelled in the period between these two publications is the rapid growth of the world-wide web and the infiltration of information technology into every aspect of our lives.

The world-wide web exerts a powerful and paradoxical influence. It has given us unparalleled access to the kind of information needed for planning clinical audits. The downside is information overload and information inflation. For example, using the term 'clinical audit', the search engine Google found 77 400 results in 0.08 seconds and Alta Vista UK retrieved 382 660 pages. The sheer volume of material is overwhelming.

The other key issue is quality control. How much of this material is worth retrieving and appraising? Health is particularly vulnerable to the triple Information Age vices of misinformation, disinformation, and outdated information.

This section sets out a framework for using the world-wide web as a means of online learning.

Planning to use the world-wide web

Few people have unlimited time or unlimited access to the Internet. What is required is swift access to the most appropriate information. Every user coming to the Internet to find information relevant to clinical audit needs to be equipped with a strategy to make the most of the medium.

Before going online, some planning is needed.

- What type of information is required?
- Where are the most likely sources?
- Can the information retrieved be relied on?

In order to address these issues, it is necessary to develop:

- questions that focus the information requirements
- awareness of available resources
- an understanding of the types of information and their uses.

Developing an awareness of likely sources of useful information

The first essential is to be able to locate information. The table below lists some questions that often come up when planning a clinical audit, and connects them to likely sources of information.

Question	Likely source
Where can I go to find clinical for guidelines?	NICE, National electronic Library Health guidelines database, National Guideline Clearinghouse (USA), SIGN
Where can I go to find criteria for clinical audit?	Clinical guidelines, performance indicators
Where can I go to find service standards?	National Service Frameworks National Centre for Health Outcomes Development Specialist Health Services Commission for Wales (SHSCW)
Which organisations have information about clinical audit?	Royal Colleges and other professional bodies
Where can I find examples of clinical audits?	Bibliographic databases
Where else can I go to get advice?	Newsgroups and other quality improvement networks

The map on page 76 and the information that follows it give an overview of clinical audit-related resources that are likely to point to relevant material. This is an important step in managing the amount of material available.

Recognising the nature and uses of information types

The proliferation of sources means increased frustration and wasted effort, unless the different types of information can be discriminated and what they have to offer is understood.

The map of resources has been divided up into sections.

- The first section looks at publications that are likely to influence clinical decision-making – clinical guidelines and systematic reviews.
- The next section looks at the related area of standard setting for services and where these are found.
- The area entitled *Sharing know-how* covers a range of information types. The stated purpose of each of these resources is to provide actual examples of quality improvement initiatives. This might take the form of projects collected in searchable databases or accessing people through discussion groups.
- *Assessing the impact* cites resources to help document and define clinical audit projects and programmes of work.

Each of these sections is only a partial foundation to the resources available. For further resources it is preferable to use specialist gateways such as OMNI and NMAP that are developed using explicit evaluation criteria.

Critical appraisal

Developing an awareness of where things are and familiarity with the different types of information available go hand-in-hand with the need to adopt a critical attitude to the information retrieved. One way of doing this is to develop specific evaluation criteria.

Criterion	Focus on
Context	Scope, audience, authority
Content	Coverage, currency, valid alternatives
Access	Usability

The websites included in this guide have been assessed against these criteria. The descriptions of each resource have been written to give as much information as possible about the context and content of each site. Where there are issues about usability, such as the need to register before gaining access to material or download software in order to read documents, this has been made explicit.

Internet resources for clinical audit

Please note that, while every effort has been made to ensure that the Internet addresses in this section (and in the book as a whole) are correct at the time of press, some may change over time.

A map of useful resources for clinical audit

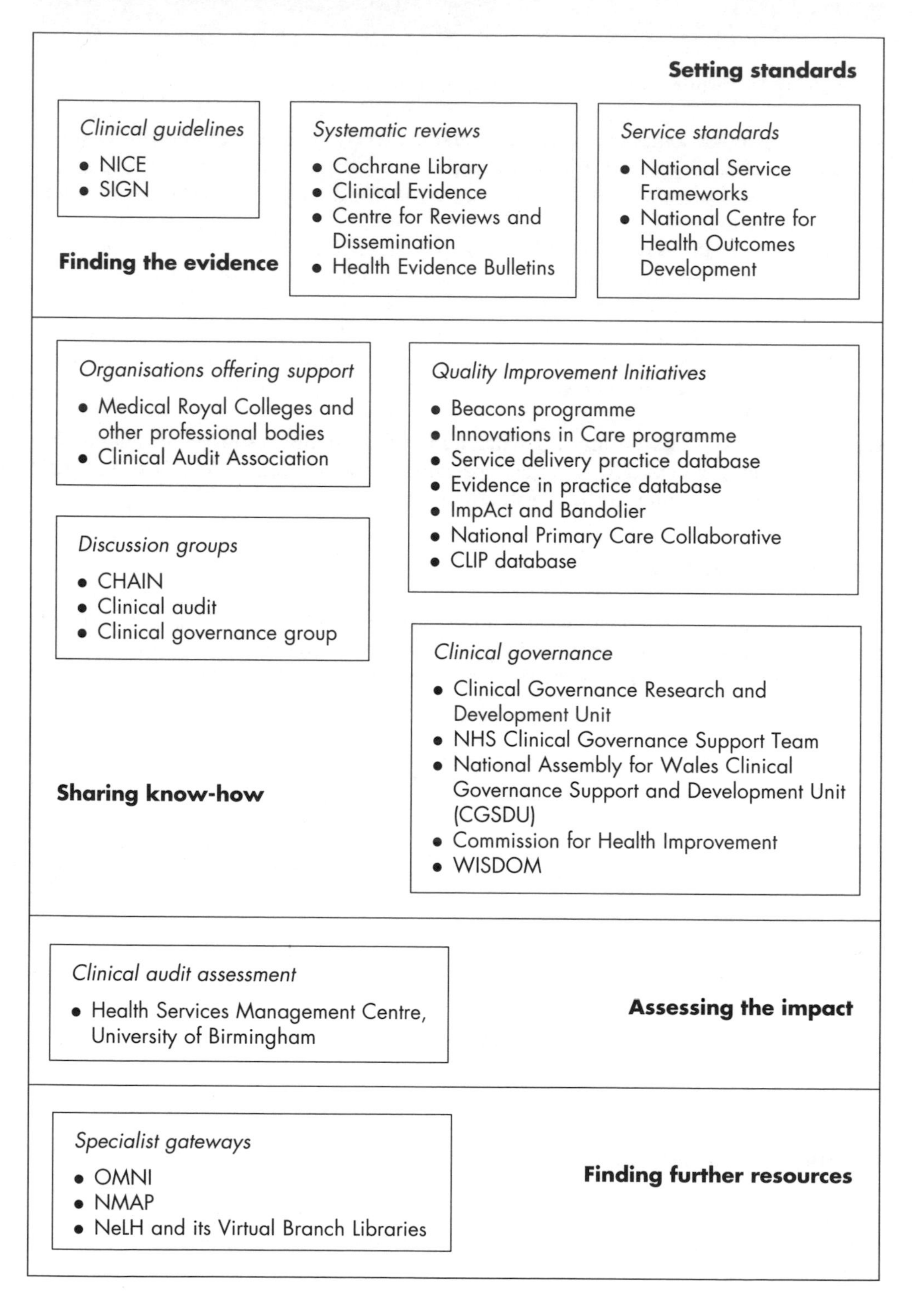

Clinical guidelines

National electronic Library for Health (NeLH) clinical guidelines database

- www.nelh.nhs.uk/guidelines_database.asp

The NeLH provides a database of evidence-based guidelines. These include guidelines from NICE and professional bodies such as the Royal College of Nursing.

National Guideline Clearing House (NGC)

- www.guideline.gov/index.asp

The NGC provides a searchable database of clinical practice guidelines. Guidelines posted on the NGC site meet several criteria including having been published in the past five years, are written in English and are based on a systematic literature search of existing scientific evidence published in peer reviewed journals. The NHC is sponsored by the Agency for Healthcare Research and Quality in partnership with the American Medical Association of Health Plans.

National Institute for Clinical Excellence (NICE)

- www.nice.org.uk

NICE is a Special Health Authority for England and Wales that provides patients, health professionals, and the public with authoritative, robust, and reliable guidance on current best practice. The guidance covers individual health technologies (including medicines, medical devices, diagnostic techniques, and procedures) and the clinical management of specific conditions.

The site includes:

- technical and summary reports of guidelines commissioned by NICE
- health technology appraisals
- referral practice guidelines.

These are available in PDF format and can be viewed with Adobe Acrobat software, which is easily downloaded from the Internet.

Scottish Intercollegiate Guideline Network (SIGN)

- www.sign.ac.uk

SIGN is a network of clinicians and healthcare professionals including representatives of all the UK Royal Medical Colleges as well as nursing, pharmacy, dentistry, and professions allied to medicine. Its objective is to improve the effectiveness and efficiency of clinical care for patients in Scotland by developing, publishing, and disseminating guidelines that identify and promote good clinical practice.

The site includes technical and summary reports of guidelines commissioned by SIGN. These are available in PDF format and can be viewed with Adobe Acrobat software, which is easily downloaded from the Internet.

Systematic reviews and critically appraised topics

Clinical Evidence

- www.clinicalevidence.com

This compendium of evidence on the effects of common clinical interventions is drawn from systematic reviews and randomised controlled trials. Each section presents a concise account of what is known and/or not known about prevention and treatment of a wide range of clinical conditions. Clinical Evidence is published by the BMJ Publishing Group. If you are an NHS employee you can register with the National electronic Library for Health (NeLH) to gain access to the full text online version.

Cochrane Library

- www.update-software.com/clibhome/clib.htm

The Cochrane Library is published quarterly on CD-ROM and the Internet, and is distributed on a subscription basis. The Abstracts of Cochrane Reviews are available without charge and can be browsed or searched. The Library consists of:

- the Cochrane Database of Systematic Reviews (regularly updated reviews of the effects of healthcare)
- Database of Abstracts of Reviews of Effectiveness (critical assessments and structured abstracts of good systematic reviews published elsewhere)
- the Cochrane Controlled Trials Register (bibliographic information on controlled trials and other sources of information on the science of reviewing research and evidence-based healthcare).

The Cochrane Library is one of several databases available to staff working in the NHS via the NeLH. Registering via an NHSnet connection is the quickest method. A password is obtained by applying online or by mail, after NHS employee status has been verified.

Centre for Reviews and Dissemination (CRD)

- www.york.ac.uk/inst/crd

CRD is a facility commissioned by the NHS Research and Development Division. It aims to identify results of good-quality health research and actively disseminate the findings to key decision-makers and consumers. It publishes the findings of systematic reviews of specific topics in the Effective Healthcare Bulletins series. The site includes full online access to all CRD publications including the Effective Healthcare Bulletin series in PDF format and can be viewed with Adobe Acrobat software, which is easily downloaded from the Internet.

Health Evidence Bulletins Wales

- www.uwcm.ac.uk/uwcm/lb/pep

The Bulletins are the result of a collaboration between the National Assembly for Wales, the Wales Office of Research and Development, the Welsh Health Authorities, health professionals from primary and secondary care in the UK, and the Department of Information Services at the University of Wales College of Medicine. Each Health Evidence Bulletin provides an overview of a subject area via succinct, current, and reliable summaries of the best evidence across a broad range of evidence types and subject areas. Full details of the supporting evidence are provided, and an increasing number of links to these publications are now available on the website.

Setting standards

National Service Frameworks web page

- www.doh.gov.uk/nsf/nsfhome.htm

National Service Frameworks (NSFs) will:

- set national standards and define service models for a specific service or care group
- put in place programmes to support implementation
- establish performance measures against which progress within an agreed timescale will be measured.

Each NSF will be developed with the assistance of an expert reference group, which will bring together health professionals, service users and carers, health service managers, partner agencies, and others.

The site includes full versions of each NSF in PDF format, which can be viewed with Adobe Acrobat software, easily downloaded from the Internet.

National Centre for Health Outcomes Development (NCHOD)

- www.ihs.ox.ac.uk/nchod

NCHOD is based jointly at the Institute of Health Sciences, University of Oxford, and the London School of Hygiene and Tropical Medicine. As part of its remit to develop defined statistical measures about clinical outcomes, NCHOD has published a number of documents on a range of conditions including asthma, breast cancer, diabetes, and stroke.

The website offers PDF versions of publications from NCHOD, which can be viewed with Adobe Acrobat software, easily downloaded from the Internet.

Sharing know-how

Bandolier

- www.jr2.ox.ac.uk/bandolier

This monthly publication aims to make knowledge and evidence from research more readily known and used. It concentrates on simplifying the results of research and presenting them accessibly to busy clinicians and patients.

The site is organised around specialist subsite collections, such as asthma and cardiac care. In addition, the whole site can be searched and the current issue viewed.

Cancer Services Collaborative

- www.nhs.uk/nationalplan/npch14.htm

The Cancer Services Collaborative Patient Pathway Programme is a major initiative to improve the quality of cancer services in England. Launched in late 1999, the 18-month programme is being piloted by nine cancer networks (one in each region and two in London). Attention is being given to breast, colorectal, lung, ovarian, and prostate cancer services. The objective is to optimise service delivery from the patient's perspective to support effective clinical care. Particular attention is being given to:

- coordinating the patient's cancer journey
- improving the patient's/carer's experience
- optimising care delivery
- matching capacity and demand.

CLIP database

- www.eguidelines.co.uk/clip/clip_main.htm

The CLIP database contains summaries of completed or ongoing local clinical effectiveness initiatives contributed by staff across the NHS. Each record presents contact details for further information. New users must register with eGuidelines to access the database; registration is free of charge. eGuidelines is part of the Medendium Group Publishing Limited.

Commission for Health Improvement (CHI)

- www.doh.gov.uk/chi/index.htm

CHI works at a local and national level to monitor and improve clinical care throughout England and Wales.

- Locally, it inspects clinical governance arrangements through clinical governance reviews, and conducts investigations or inquiries into serious service failures.
- Nationally, CHI undertakes studies reviewing the implementation of the National Service Frameworks, guidance from the National Institute for Clinical Excellence and other NHS priorities.
- CHI also has a role in providing leadership for spreading good practice in clinical governance.

The site covers the range of CHI activities including details of Clinical Governance Reviews. It publishes the programme of reviews, information on the review process, review results and work on the National Service Frameworks.

ImpAct

- www.jr2.ox.ac.uk/bandolier/ImpAct/index.html

ImpAct is a publication that focuses on ways of raising standards and improving the delivery of services to patients. It identifies ways of improving performance which have been successful and which are transferable. Reports will include successful local initiatives and material developed locally that could be adapted for use elsewhere.

ImpAct focuses on:

- clinical governance and questions about clinical quality, such as the application of National Service Frameworks, emergency pressures, demand, and waiting times
- integration of services across institutional boundaries
- primary care groups and questions about service delivery
- involving patients and the public
- developments in human resources such as staffing and skill mix issues.

Criteria for guiding choice of initiatives include:

- availability of information to describe the benefits to patients and organisations
- transferability and general applicability of projects to other situations
- affordability of projects within normal budgets.

The site includes a searchable archive of back numbers, and a PDF version of the current issue, which can be viewed with Adobe Acrobat software, easily downloaded from the Internet.

Institute for Healthcare Improvement (IHI)

- www.ihi.org

IHI is a Boston-based, independent, non-profit organisation that has worked since 1991 to accelerate improvement in healthcare systems in the USA, Canada, and Europe, by fostering collaboration among healthcare organisations.

The site gives details of conferences, courses and project work. Certain resources are available online, including a publication on reducing medical errors under the IHI patient safety resources homepage, which is available as a PDF file that can be viewed with Adobe Acrobat software, easily downloaded from the Internet.

National Co-ordinating Centre for NHS Service Delivery and Organisation (NCCSDO) research and development programme

- www.sdo.lshtm.ac.uk

The NCCSDO research and development programme is a national research programme established to consolidate and develop the evidence base on the organisation, management and delivery of healthcare services.

The site contains publications including two on managing change in the NHS:

- *Organisational Change. A Review for Health Care Managers, Professionals and Researchers* – a review of models of change management to help managers, professionals and researchers find their way around the literature and consider the evidence available about different approaches to change
- a summary version called *Making Informed Decisions on Change. Key Points for Health Care Managers and Professionals.*

NHS Beacons programme

- www.nhsbeacons.org.uk

The Beacon programme was established to underpin the spread of good practice across the service. Beacon status is awarded to those organisations offering patients access to 'faster, more convenient and more appropriate care'. The areas highlighted so far include:

- outpatient services
- coronary heart disease
- stroke
- palliative care
- human resources
- health improvement
- mental health
- personality disorder.

The site provides a database of Beacon sites and their schemes. This is searchable by key area (e.g. primary care), text phrase, topic, dissemination activity, or NHS region. Dates when the Beacon sites can be visited can also be found.

The Innovations in Care Programme in the National Assembly for Wales is running a similar programme in Wales.

NHS Learning Zone

- www.doh.gov.uk/learningzone/index.htm

The purpose of the Learning Zone is to share information about how NHS and non-NHS organisations have tried to improve service delivery for patients. It houses several facilities aimed at helping people learn from others about the best ways of improving service delivery and management. It hosts information about the Beacons programme, training programmes for management, benchmarking, and other resources. Links to external databases are available (note that some links will not be available to users who do not have NHSnet access).

National Patient Safety Agency

- www.npsa.org.uk

The National Patient Safety Agency is responsible for designing and implementing a system for reporting adverse events involving NHS patients. The site provides information about the development of the system. In addition it offers a range of other resources including alerts (e.g. administering vincristine), a library of briefings and presentations, research, news, events, and message boards for professional groups.

National Primary Care Development Team

- www.npdt.org

The National Primary Care Development Team (NPDT) has been set up to deliver the Government's modernisation agenda in primary care by using a specific technique called a 'collaborative'. This method was developed by the Institute for Healthcare Improvement (*see* page 81) in the USA and has been applied to other healthcare settings to achieve rapid and sustainable improvement. The National Primary Care Collaborative brings together invited Primary Care Groups/Primary Care Trusts to improve the overall experience and clinical outcomes for patients by sharing innovative ideas that have been proved to work, through collating best practice and bringing innovators together with quality experts to develop an implementation package.

The site gives full details of the project including the methodology used, the proposed timetable of events, and contact details of the NPDT and regional contacts.

Our Healthier Nation in Practice (OHNiP) database

- www.ohn.gov.uk/database/database.htm

The OHNiP database holds records describing a range of projects and initiatives contributing to the aims of *Saving Lives: Our Healthier Nation* (i.e. tackling health inequalities). The site includes the OHN database and links to online journals and databases, statistical sources, professional groups and organisations, and mailing lists.

Service Delivery Practice Database

- www.doh.gov.uk/learningzone/sdpinter.htm

This is a database of projects undertaken by NHS individuals and organisations. It is published on NHSNet only.

Advice on clinical audit – discussion groups

Contacts, Help, Advice, Information Network (C.H.A.I.N.)

- www.open.gov.uk/doh/ntrd/chain/chain.htm

C.H.A.I.N. is a network bringing together healthcare professionals, librarians, teachers, and researchers interested in evidence-based practice. C.H.A.I.N. is now managed by London Region's research and development programme, but is being developed as a national resource for the NHS.

Details of how to join the network are available on the website. The database of contacts is available free of charge on the Internet, CD-ROM, and floppy disk. The Internet version allows online data entry and searches.

Clinical-governance-group

- www.mailbase.ac.uk/lists/clinical-governance-group

This self-selected group of health professionals who wish to discuss, share, and learn about clinical governance issues is a subset of C.H.A.I.N.

The site explains how to register with the discussion list, post a message to the list, or review previous messages by date or theme.

Organisations offering support for clinical audit and clinical governance

Clinical Audit Association (CAA)

- www.the-caa-ltd.demon.co.uk

Originally founded in 1991, CAA is a membership organisation open to everyone with an interest in improving the quality of healthcare through clinical audit. Major aims include:

- to promote clinical audit as a vehicle for the improvement of patient care
- to promote a high standard of practice by clinical audit professionals
- to facilitate the professional development in clinical audit of members of the Association
- to provide a forum for the acquisition and dissemination of information related to the development of clinical audit and to promote the professional interests of members in matters relating to training, qualifications and terms and conditions of service.

Clinical Governance Association (CGA)
- www.bamm.co.uk/CGA Website – Home.html

The CGA is a membership association set up to provide a support network for staff whose primary role is to lead or assist with the implementation of clinical governance across the health economy. It provides training and development programmes, forums for problem solving and opportunities for skill sharing.

Clinical Governance Research and Development Unit (CGRDU)
- www.le.ac.uk/cgrdu/index.html

CGRDU came into existence on 1 April 1999, succeeding the Eli Lilly National Clinical Audit Centre, which since 1992 had been a national resource in the field of clinical audit, particularly in the setting of primary healthcare and at the interface between primary and secondary care. The principal function of CGRDU is research and development within the emerging field of clinical governance. The site includes audit protocols to view and download.

Clinical Governance Support and Development Unit (Wales) (CGSDU)
Website is under development at time of press, but will be accessible via www.wales.gov.uk/.

The CGSDU was established in April 2001 to provide leadership and support to the NHS to develop, strengthen, and improve clinical governance in Wales. Its programme of work includes:

- a Board Support Programme: creating the vision of what clinical governance should look like, integrating the component parts, spreading across the whole organisation in a multiprofessional way, incorporating cross-sector and public/patient views
- a Clinical Governance Development Programme: to support clinical team working aimed at implementation of priority areas (e.g. NSFs, clinical networks)
- a Clinical Governance Learning Network: supporting clinical governance leads, facilitators, and others to identify, develop, and disseminate useful tools, techniques etc.
- direct training and information
- work with NHS organisations in specific areas: e.g. implementing CHI recommendations, progressing activity against clinical governance performance measures.

Clinical Resource and Audit Group (CRAG)
- www.show.scot.nhs.uk/crag

CRAG is the lead body within the Scottish Executive Health Department, promoting clinical effectiveness in Scotland. The main committee of CRAG, together with its subcommittees, provides advice to the Health Department, acts as a national forum to support and facilitate the implementation of the clinical effectiveness agenda, and funds a number of clinical effectiveness programmes and projects.

The site incorporates key documents on clinical effectiveness, including a national initiative about the management of diabetes.

Clinical Governance resources – Library and Information Service, Health Services Management Centre, University of Birmingham

- spp3.bham.ac.uk/hsmc/library/hot_topic_clinicalgov.htm

The Library and Information Service incorporates the collections and resources of the Health Services Management Centre Library and the West Midlands NHS Executive Library.

The site includes a collection of clinical governance resources under a 'Hot Topics' section, bringing together material from around the NHS health regions.

NHS Clinical Governance Support Team

- www.cgsupport.org

The NHS Clinical Governance Support Team has been created to help deliver the successful implementation of clinical governance 'on the ground'. The aim is to support the delivery of high-quality, patient-centred healthcare that is accountable, systematic, and sustainable.

WISDOM

- www.wisdomnet.co.uk

The WISDOM project delivers networked professional development for primary health care, using Internet technologies for information sharing and communication. The project contains resources about clinical governance and quality assurance, as well as evidence-based practice, Primary Care Group organisation, and change management. The WISDOM Centre is based at the Institute of General Practice and Primary Care, Community Sciences Centre, Northern General Hospital, Sheffield.

The site runs a number of 'virtual conferences', discussion groups for networked professional learning. These include a group for clinical governance and clinical updates. The site contains an extensive library of online resources relevant to primary healthcare, including the Resource Pack for Clinical Governance.

Selection of Medical Royal Colleges and professional bodies

College of Occupational Therapists – Clinical Audit

- www.cot.co.uk

The British Association and College of Occupational Therapists is a trade union and professional association.

The site provides information on:

- publications about audit
- a database of audits completed by occupational therapists that is used to facilitate networking
- workshops and study days
- participation in relevant national audits
- clinical guideline development.

Community Practitioners and Health Visitors Association (CPHVA)
- www.msfcphva.org/index1.html

CPHVA is the UK professional body that represents registered nurses and health visitors who work in a primary or community health setting.

The site gives details of CPHVA publications including a clinical effectiveness resource pack and links to systematic reviews relevant to the profession.

Joint Royal Colleges Ambulance Liaison Committee (JRCALC)
- www.asancep.org.uk/JRCALC

The JRCALC was created in 1989 to provide a focus for the UK Ambulance Service in its interactions with other professional healthcare groups.

The site provides:

- information about a number of quality improvement initiatives, including a national clinical audit of acute myocardial infarction by ambulance services
- updates on the work of the clinical guidelines sub-committee and its work in developing pre-hospital guidelines.

Royal College of Anaesthetists
- www.rcoa.ac.uk

The College has produced a guide for departments of anaesthesia summarising the methods by which the medical profession is currently regulated, and gives guidance to anaesthetists about how departments of anaesthesia can set, maintain, and monitor standards of good practice within this changing environment. The College has also established an ongoing national reporting system for recording critical incidents and sharing information about such incidents on a national basis.

The professional standards section of the site includes such College publications as *Raising the Standard: a Compendium of Audit Recipes for Continuous Improvement in Anaesthesia* and information about the College's critical incident reporting scheme. All online versions are available as PDF files, which can be viewed using Adobe Acrobat software, easily downloaded from the Internet.

Royal College of General Practitioners (RCGP) – Clinical Practice Evaluation Programme (CPEP)

- www.shef.ac.uk/~scharr/publich/cpep/index.html

CPEP forms part of the RCGP Quality Initiative. It is a new, professionally led, multi-level, practical evaluation system to enable all general practice teams to evaluate and compare the quality of their care through a process of minimum data collection, comparison, and feedback relating to appropriate evidence-based review criteria.

The site provides further details of the initiative, including evidence-based review criteria of coronary heart disease, adults with asthma, and type 2 diabetes (foot care). These are available in PDF format which can be viewed with Adobe Acrobat software, easily downloaded from the Internet.

Royal College of Nursing (RCN) – Quality Improvement Programme

- www.rcn.org.uk

The Quality Improvement Programme incorporates educational, networking, research, and developmental activities in the areas of clinical effectiveness, clinical guidelines, and quality. The Quality Improvement Network promotes information sharing between nurses interested or involved in promoting quality through 11 regional groups that organise regular meetings and seminars. Membership of the network is free to all RCN members. Research focuses primarily on evaluating quality improvement and audit and, to this end, a number of studies have been completed which look at the impact on clinical practice and patient outcomes. The programme is taking the lead in the RCN's clinical effectiveness strategy. Current work includes the development of nurse-led clinical guidelines and implementation of guidelines in practice. The Information Service supports nurses and midwives in the UK who want to ensure that the care they provide is clinically effective.

The site includes access to RCN clinical guideline publications, available as PDF files which can be viewed with Adobe Acrobat software, easily downloaded from the Internet.

Royal College of Obstetricians and Gynaecologists

- www.rcog.org.uk

The Effectiveness Support Unit is a multidisciplinary team which includes clinicians and midwives, as well as those with expertise in methodology, statistics, epidemiology, and medical informatics. The Good Medical Practice section of the site includes clinical practice guidelines produced by the College. It also includes online versions of *Effective Procedures in Maternity Care Suitable for Audit* and a similar publication on gynaecological procedures.

Royal College of Pathologists – Clinical Audit and Effectiveness Unit

- www.rcpath.org

The Unit aims to offer support and advice to medical staff, clinical scientists, medical laboratory scientific officers, and audit support staff wishing to undertake clinical audit in pathology. The unit holds a database of audit projects submitted by trusts and regional groups from around the UK. Searches, by clinical topic or keywords, can be performed by the Audit Department. The database is available as a catalogue of titles sorted by specialty and is updated twice a year. The Unit also conducts workshops on clinical audit in pathology for medical and laboratory staff, and is intended to impart practical advice and ideas for carrying out effective audit.

The site covers national audit projects, details on accessing the audit projects database, and engaging in clinical audit training.

Royal College of Physicians of England Clinical Effectiveness and Evaluation Unit (CEEU)

- www.rcplondon.ac.uk/college/ceeu

The aims of the CEEU are:

- to facilitate the development of evidence-based guidelines
- to devise and validate measurement tools for assessing best practice and clinical outcome indicators of the management of patient care.

Online reports include a clinical guideline for stroke and data sets for myocardial infarction and lung cancer.

Royal College of Psychiatrists Research Unit (CRU)

- www.rcpsych.ac.uk/cru

CRU works in three identified areas:

- mental health service research
- quality improvement
- informatics.

An emphasis on 'getting research into practice' underpins the work of the Unit, which works to put its findings into practice. Examples include the production of clinical practice guidelines, organising national clinical audit projects, supporting the use of outcome measures, and the provision of information to support mental health services in increasing their effectiveness.

The site provides updates on current projects and completed projects, publications and forthcoming training events and conferences.

Royal College of Radiologists

- www.rcr.ac.uk

The Royal College of Radiologists is concerned with standards in the medical specialties of clinical radiology (diagnostic imaging) and clinical oncology (cancer treatment).

The site has a section on the audit activities of the College, including online access to several publications containing information about a national audit of waiting times for radiotherapy. The college has also published evidence-based guidelines on the management of lung cancer, prostate cancer, breast cancer, generic radiotherapy, and testicular cancer. These are available in HTML, PDF, and MS Word 6.0 formats. Adobe Acrobat software is required to view PDF files. The College has also produced information leaflets for patients undergoing various radiology procedures. These are available in HTML and MS Word formats.

Royal College of Surgeons of England – Clinical Effectiveness Unit (CEU)

- www.rcseng.ac.uk/ceu/default.asp

The CEU is a collaboration between the College and the Health Services Research Unit at the London School of Hygiene & Tropical Medicine.

The site describes the activities of the CEU.

Royal Pharmaceutical Society (RPSGB) Clinical Audit Unit

- www.rpsgb.org.uk/audhome.htm

The RPSGB Clinical Audit Unit has a remit to develop audit throughout pharmacy and has developed audits covering most of pharmacy practice. The unit can provide training in clinical audit for pharmacists, ranging from simple lectures about audit to full-day courses aimed at either novices or more experienced pharmacists.

The site features clinical audit templates from the Pharmacy Audit Support Pack available as PDF files, which can be viewed with Adobe Acrobat software, easily downloaded from the Internet.

Evaluating Clinical Audit

The clinical audit assessment framework – Health Services Management Centre, University of Birmingham

- http://www.hsmc3.bham.ac.uk/hsmc/publicns/caaf.htm

The information pack that can be downloaded from this website describes an approach to assessing and improving the effectiveness of clinical audit activities. It was developed by the Health Services Management Centre at the University of Birmingham for the NHS Executive.

The site includes online versions of:

- an introduction to the framework and how it can be used by health authorities, NHS trusts, audit groups, and individual health professionals in assessing and then improving their own clinical audit activities
- forms that have been developed to help in using the clinical audit assessment framework. They offer sample reporting formats for monitoring clinical audit activities and checklists for assessing and then taking action to improve audit projects and programmes
- completed examples of these forms, to provide an idea of how they can be used by different organisations and in different settings
- full text of a report that describes the clinical audit assessment framework in considerable detail. It is intended to act as a reference and source of further information, offering specific guidance on use of the framework in different settings, and including a detailed definition of the framework.

Gateways

Organising Medical Networked Information (OMNI) and Nursing, Midwifery and Allied Health Professionals Gateway (NMAP)

- www.omni.ac.uk
- nmap.ac.uk

OMNI offers free access to a searchable catalogue of Internet sites covering health and medicine. Each record appearing on the OMNI/NMAP site has been evaluated and checked against explicit criteria. The site is hosted and managed by the University of Nottingham. NMAP focuses on material relating to nursing, midwifery, and allied health professionals. NMAP is a collaboration between Nottingham and the University of Sheffield and the Royal College of Nursing. Users can search OMNI/NMAP, or select one of the other BIOME gateways to find Internet resources in other areas of the life sciences. Records can be viewed in a number of ways, such as by resource type or by browsing records clustered under National Library of Medicine headings. Other facilities offered include an online tutorial about searching and using medical sites on the Internet called the Internet Medic (www.omni.ac.uk/vts/medic).

National electronic Library for Health and its Virtual Branch Libraries

- www.nelh.nhs.uk

The role of the NeLH is to provide healthcare professionals and the public (through NHS Direct Online and the New Library Network) with information to support healthcare related decisions. The NeLH has also purchased licences on behalf of the NHS for databases such as the Cochrane Library of Systematic Reviews and Clinical Evidence, the BMJ publication of appraised topics. NHS staff can register for password access to these resources.

The NeLH also has Virtual Branch Libraries containing collections of information about a specific aspect of health, or a particular disease or condition. Each collection is put together by specialists in that particular field and scrutinised by their peers.

The NeLH contains portals presenting information relevant to a particular professional group, such as nurses, midwives, and allied health professions.

The nursing portal is at www.nelh.nhs.uk/nurse.

Appendix III: national audit projects sponsored by the National Institute for Clinical Excellence

Completed audit projects (1996–2000)

Title	Developed by	Key contact
The National Sentinel Audit of Stroke	Clinical Effectiveness and Evaluation Unit on behalf of the Intercollegiate Stroke Working Party Royal College of Physicians of London 11 St Andrews Place London NW1 4LE	P Irwin Tel: 0207 935 1174 Email: ceeu@rcplondon.ac.uk
The National Collaborative Audit for the Management of Elderly People Who Have Fallen	Chartered Society of Physiotherapy and College of Occupational Therapists	Rowena Clarke 14 Bedford Row London WC1R 4ED Tel: 0207 306 6632 Email: clarker@cphysio.org.uk
National Sentinel Audit Toolkit for Acute Back Pain	Institute for Musculoskeletal Research and Clinical Implementation 13–15 Parkwood Road Bournemouth BH5 2DF	Alan Breen Tel: 01202 436 275 Email: imrci.abreen@aecc.ac.uk
The National Sentinel Audit of the Management of Violence in Mental Health Settings	Royal College of Psychiatrists 6th Floor, 83 Victoria Street London SW1H 0HW	Kim McLellan Tel: 0207 227 0839 Email: kim.mclellan@virgin.net

National Sentinel Audit Pilot Project for the Management of Patients With Venous Leg Ulcers	Royal College of Nursing Available from: RCN Publishing Company Ltd Tel: 01275 847180	Ross Scrivener/ Lesley Overall Information Services, RCN Quality Improvement Programme, Room 411, 20 Cavendish Square, London W1G 0RN Email: qip.hq@rcn.org.uk
National Sentinel Clinical Audit of Evidence Based Prescribing for Older People (EBPOP)	Clinical Effectiveness and Evaluation Unit Royal College of Physicians of London 11 St Andrews Place London NW1	R Grant Tel: 0207 935 1174 Email: ceeu@rcplondon.ac.uk
National Audit of *Helicobacter pylori* and the Management of Dyspepsia	Royal College of Pathologists 3 Carlton Terrace London SW1Y 4AF	Claire du Boulay Professional Standards Unit 2 Carlton House Terrace London SW1Y 5AF Email: PSU@rcpath.org
National Sentinel Caesarean Section Audit (available from www.rcog.org.uk)	Clinical Effectiveness Support Unit at the Royal College of Obstetricians and Gynaecologists 27 Sussex Place, Regent's Park London NW1 4RG	Jane Thomas Email: jthomas@rcog.org.uk Enquiries: NSCSA@rcog.org.uk
Clinical Practice Evaluation Programme (CPEP)	Royal College of General Practitioners 14 Princes Gate, Hyde Park London SW7 1PU	Aileen McIntosh Email: A.Mcintosh@sheffield.ac.uk
National Sentinel Cataract Audit	Royal College of Ophthalmologists	Parul Desai Moorfields Eye Hospital City Road London EC1V 2PD Email: parul.desai@moorfields.nhs.uk

Audit projects ongoing at the time of press

Title	Developed by	Key contact	Expected publication date
Sudden Unexpected Death in Epilepsy (SUDEP)	Epilepsy Bereaved	Jane Hanna Tel: 01235 772 850 Email: epilepsybereaved@dial.pipex.com	May 2002
Myocardial Infarction National Audit Project (MINAP)	Clinical Effectiveness and Evaluation Unit on behalf of the MINAP Steering Group Royal College of Physicians 11 St Andrews Place London NW1 4LE	L Walker Tel: 0207 935 1174 Email: ceeu@rcplondon.ac.uk	Dec 2002
Quality Indicators for Diabetes Services (QUIDS)	Diabetes UK 10 Queen Anne Street London W1M 0BD	Moira Murphy Email: alexis@diabetes.org.uk	Sept 2002
Continence	National Collaborating Centre for Chronic Conditions c/o Royal College of Physicians 11 St Andrews Place London NW1 4LE	J Ingham Email: jane.ingham@rcplondon.ac.uk	2003/4
Parenteral Nutrition in Pre-term Infants	National Collaborating Centre for Women and Children c/o Royal College of Obstetricians and Gynaecologists 27 Sussex Place, Regent's Park London NW1 4RG	Jane Thomas Email: jthomas@rcog.org.uk	March 2003
Coronary Heart Disease in Primary Care	National Collaborating Centre for Primary Care c/o Royal College of General Practitioners 14 Princes Gate, Hyde Park London SW7	Richard Baker Email: rb14@le.ac.uk	Aug 2002

Appendix IV: further reading

Compendia of audit examples

These are current at the time of press though they may, of course, be updated over time.

Godwin R, de Lacey G, Manhire A, eds. *Clinical Audit in Radiology: 100+ Recipes*. London: Royal College of Radiologists, 1996. www.rcr.ac.uk

Lack J, White L, Thoms G, Rollin A, eds. *Raising the Standard. A Compendium of Audit Recipes for Continuous Quality Improvement in Anaesthesia*. London: Royal College of Anaesthetists, 2000. www.rcoa.ac.uk/publications.asp.

Royal College of Obstetricians and Gynaecologists. *Effective Procedures in Gynaecology Suitable for Audit*. London: Royal College of Obstetricians and Gynaecologists, 1996. www.rcog.org.uk.

Royal College of Obstetricians and Gynaecologists. *Effective Procedures in Maternity Care Suitable for Audit*. London: Royal College of Obstetricians and Gynaecologists, 1996. www.rcog.org.uk.

Royal College of Paediatrics and Child Health. *Clinical Audit in Paediatrics and Child Health – Some Examples*. London: Royal College of Paediatrics and Child Health, 1997. Contents: over 30 clinical audits contributed by paediatricians working in both the acute and community sectors. www.rcpch.ac.uk.

Royal College of Physicians. *Audit of Acute Medical Admissions*. London: Royal College of Physicians, 1997. www.rcplondon.ac.uk.

Royal Pharmaceutical Society of Great Britain. *Improving Patient Care. A Team Approach. Examples of Multi-Professional Audits Involving the Community Pharmacist*. London: Royal Pharmaceutical Society of Great Britain, 1996. Contents: 10 sample clinical audits. www.rpsgb.org.uk/audhome.htm.

Overviews

Chartered Society of Physiotherapy. *Sources of Information on Clinical Audit*. London: Chartered Society of Physiotherapy, 1998. www.csp.org.uk.

College of Occupational Therapists. *Clinical Audit in Occupational Therapy. Result of a National Survey and Recommendations for Action*. London: College of Occupational Therapists, 1997. www.cot.co.uk.

College of Occupational Therapists. *Clinical Audit Information Pack*. London: College of Occupational Therapists, 1998. www.cot.co.uk.

Fraser RC, Lakhani MK, Baker RH. *Evidence-Based Audit in General Practice. From Principles to Practice*. Oxford: Butterworth-Heinemann, 1998.

Health Visitors' Association. *Adding Value. Using Clinical Audit to Develop School and Nursing Services*. Contents: the potential for school nursing; clinical audit explained; examples from practice – school health entry checks, road safety, individual counselling, asthma management, drop-in clinic. London: Health Visitors' Association, 1996. www.msfcphva.org/index1.html.

Hudson R. Quality Counts. *An Introductory Guide to Clinical Audit in Primary Health Care*. London: Health Visitors' Association, 1996. Contents: what is clinical audit?; the clinical audit process; your questions answered; examples of audit in primary care nursing; further help and information; glossary of terms. www.msfcphva.org/index1.html.

Morrell C, Harvey G. *The Clinical Audit Handbook. Improving the Quality of Health Care*. London: Baillière Tindall, 1999. www.harcourt-international.com/catalogue/title.cfm?ISBN=070202418X.

Morris M. *Midwifery Audit Good Practice Guide*. London: Royal College of Midwives, 1998. Contents: what is clinical audit; process of audit. www.rcm.org.uk.

Palmer C, Fenner J. *Getting the Message Across*. London: Royal College of Psychiatrists, 1999. www.rcpsych.ac.uk/cru.

Royal College of Anaesthetists and the Association of Anaesthetists of Great Britain and Ireland. *Good Practice. A Guide for the Departments of Anaesthesia*. London: Royal College of Anaesthetists and the Association of Anaesthetists of Great Britain and Ireland, 1998. Contents: ethical framework; leadership, management and administration; record keeping; audit; CPD/CME; poorly performing anaesthetists; the way forward. www.rcoa.ac.uk/publications.asp.

Royal College of General Practitioners. *Audit in General Practice*. London: Royal College of General Practitioners, 1996. www.rcgp.org.uk/rcgp/webmaster/quality_and_standards.asp.

Royal College of Pathologists. *Clinical Audit in Pathology*. London: Royal College of Pathologists, 1997. www.rcpath.org/activities/list.html

Royal College of Radiologists. *Clinical Governance and Revalidation. A Practical Guide for Radiologists*. London: Royal College of Radiologists, 2000. www.rcr.ac.uk.

Royal College of Speech and Language. *Communicating Quality*. London: Royal College of Speech and Language Therapists, 1996. www.rcslt.org.

Royal Pharmaceutical Society of Great Britain. *Improving Patient Care. A Team Approach. Guidance on Involving the Community Pharmacists in Multi-Professional Clinical Audit*. London: Royal Pharmaceutical Society of Great Britain, 1996. Contents: what is clinical audit?; what constitutes good audit; the team approach;

how do community pharmacists contribute to health outcomes; what prevents involvement; sources of help and advice. www.rpsgb.org.uk/audhome.htm.

Patient involvement

Kelson M. *Promoting Patient Involvement in Clinical Audit. Practical Guidance on Achieving Effective Involvement*. London: College of Health and the Clinical Outcomes Group – Patient Subgroup, 1998. Contents: why involve patients in clinical audit?; who should be involved in clinical audit?; when and how to involve patients in clinical audit; barriers to involvement and how to overcome them; checklists for all the sections. http://homepages.which.net/~collegeofhealth.

Kelson M. *A Guide to Involving Older People in Local Clinical Audit Activity: National Sentinel Audits Involving Older People*. London: College of Health, Chartered Society of Physiotherapy and Royal College of Nursing, 1999. Contents: how to involve older people in clinical audit; involving specific subgroups of older people in clinical audit – ethnic minorities, older people with physical, sensory and communication problems, older people with dementia, learning disabilities, mental health problems; developing the involvement of older people in clinical audit – organisational strategies and checklist. http://homepages.which.net/~collegeofhealth.

Specific areas

Hardman E, Joughin C. *FOCUS on Clinical Audit in Child and Adolescent Mental Health Services*. London: Royal College of Psychiatrists, 1998. www.rcpsych.ac.uk/cru.

MacLean Steel K, Palmer C. *Improving the Care of Elderly People with Mental Health Problems: Clinical Audit Project Examples*. London: Royal College of Psychiatrists, 1999. www.rcpsych.ac.uk/cru.

MacLean Steel K, Palmer C. *Improving the Care of People with Learning Disabilities: Clinical Audit Examples*. London: Royal College of Psychiatrists, 2000. www.rcpsych.ac.uk/cru.

MacLean Steel K, Palmer C. *Improving the Care of People in Substance Misuse Services: Clinical Audit Project Examples*. London: Royal College of Psychiatrists, 2000. www.rcpsych.ac.uk/cru.

Queenborough R, Pruce D. *Managing Antibiotic Prescribing. Audit Handbook*. London: National Prescribing Centre and Royal Pharmaceutical Society of Great Britain, 2000. www.rpsgb.org.uk/audhome.htm.

Royal Pharmaceutical Society of Great Britain. *Supporting Medicines Compliance. Dosage Instructions Audit. Introductory Work Book: Baseline/Pre-Audit*. London: Royal Pharmaceutical Society of Great Britain, 1998. www.rpsgb.org.uk/audhome.htm.

Royal College of Physicians. *Promoting Continence. Clinical Audit Scheme for the Management of Urinary and Faecal Incontinence*. London: Royal College of Physicians, 1998. www.rcplondon.ac.uk.

Royal College of Physicians. *The Care Scheme. Clinical Audit of Long-Term Care of Elderly People*. London: Royal College of Physicians, 1999. www.rcplondon.ac.uk.

Royal College of Physicians. *National Sentinel Audit for Stroke – a Tool for Raising Standards of Care*. London: Royal College of Physicians, 1999. www.rcplondon.ac.uk.

Appendix V: key points and key notes

Stage One: preparing for audit

Key points

- Clinical audit is used to improve aspects of care in a wide variety of topics. It is also used in association with changes in systems of care, or to confirm that current practice meets the expected level of performance.
- Clinical audit projects are best conducted within a structured programme, with effective leadership, participation by all staff, and an emphasis on team working and support.
- Organisations must recognise that clinical audit requires appropriate funding.
- Organisations need to recognise that improvements in care resulting from clinical audit can increase costs.
- The participation of staff in selecting topics enables concerns about care to be reported and addressed. Participation in choice of topic is not always necessary, but may have a role in reducing resistance to change.
- The priorities of those receiving care can differ quite markedly from those of clinicians. Service users should therefore be involved in the clinical audit process.
- There are practical approaches for user involvement in all stages of audit, including the design, the collection of data about performance, and in implementing change.
- Organisations should ensure that their healthcare staff learn the skills of clinical audit.
- The most frequently cited barrier to successful clinical audit is the failure of organisations to provide sufficient protected time for healthcare teams.
- Those involved in organising audit programmes must consider various methods of engaging the full participation of all health service staff.

Stage Two: selecting criteria

Key points

- Clinical audit can include assessment of the process and/or outcome of care. The choice depends on the topic and objectives of the audit.
- Explicit rather than implicit criteria should be preferred.
- Systematic methods should be used to derive criteria from evidence. These include methods for deriving criteria from good-quality guidelines or from reviews of the evidence.
- Criteria should relate to important aspects of care and be measurable.
- Provided that research evidence confirms that clinical care processes have an influence on outcome, measurement of the process of care is generally more sensitive and provides a direct measure of the quality of care.
- Measurement of outcome can be used to identify problems in care, provided outcomes are clear, influenced by process, and occur within a short period.
- Adjustment for case mix is generally required for comparing the outcomes of different providers.
- If the criteria incorporate, or are based on, the views of professionals or other groups, formal consensus methods are preferable.
- There is insufficient evidence to determine whether it is necessary to set target levels of performance in audit. However, reference to levels achieved in audits undertaken by other professionals is useful.
- In some audits, benchmarking techniques could help participants in audit to avoid setting unnecessarily low or unrealistically high target levels of performance.

Stage Three: measuring level of performance

Key points

- Patient registers are used to identify patients, but registers can be incomplete. The identification of patients using several sources can be an appropriate response.
- Although clinical records are frequently used as the source of data, they are often incomplete. The collection of data from several sources can help to overcome this problem.
- When collecting data, a carefully developed data abstraction tool is recommended. Training data abstractors can improve data consistency.
- If routinely collected data are available, they may be appropriate for use in audit.

- Electronic information systems can contribute to audit in many ways, including: improving access to research evidence; identifying users; collecting data; prompting change through record templates; and enabling revised systems of care to be introduced.

Key notes

- Health service professionals must be aware of the ethical implications of audit and their responsibilities under the Data Protection Act (1998) when collecting data and presenting results.
- Every audit should define the users to be included, the aspects of care under review, and the time period over which the criteria apply.
- Health service professionals need to be able to apply appropriate sampling techniques.

Stage Four: making improvements

Key points

- A systematic approach to implementation appears to be more effective. Such an approach includes the identification of local barriers to change, the support of teamwork, and the use of a variety of specific methods.
- An investigation of potential barriers to change assists in the development of implementation plans.
- Teams undertaking audit that are appropriately supported and able to use a variety of techniques can identify potential barriers and develop practical implementation plans.
- Contextual factors influence the likelihood of change. These include the significance of change to service users, the effectiveness of teamwork, and the organisational environment.
- Those planning audits should avoid relying on feedback alone as the method of implementing change; although feedback of data alone can occasionally be effective, change is much more likely if it forms part of a more complex set of change processes/interventions.
- The dissemination of educational materials, such as guidelines, has little effect unless accompanied by the use of selected implementation methods.
- Interactive educational interventions including outreach, service user and/or professional reminders (whether manual or computerised), decision support, and system changes can sometimes, but not always, be effective.
- In audit, the use of multifaceted interventions chosen to suit the particular circumstances is more likely to be effective in changing performance than the use of a single intervention alone.

Key note

- Clinical governance programmes offer a structure to support efforts to make improvements, including personal professional development, support of teams, and clear accountability.

Stage Five: sustaining improvement

Key points

- Organisations can use recognised assessment techniques to evaluate the quality of audit carried out by healthcare professionals.
- Alternative models of assessing healthcare provision, such as delay pattern analysis and critical incident review, can assist with identifying and investigating certain deficiencies in care. The most effective approaches for ensuring that these methods lead to improved care are uncertain.

Key notes

- Improvement in care implemented as a part of clinical audit must be monitored, evaluated, sustained, and reinforced within a supportive environment.
- Structures and systems must be developed to enable organisations to integrate improvements within a planned strategy.
- A culture is required that makes the user's experience the primary motivation for improvements, creates confident staff who do not fear reporting or confronting inadequate performance, and has clear and constant objectives.
- Systems, structures, and specific mechanisms are available for monitoring sustained improvement.

Appendix VI: checklists

In the checklists that follow, the assessment points are derived from the key points and key notes. In reviewing an audit project or audit programme, it must be determined whether the project or programme accords with the assessment points. The checklists are intended to be used as an aid to improving audit projects and programmes, and should not be applied as a definitive or inflexible yardstick. It should also be noted that some items will not apply to all audits. The checklists may also be used as an aid when planning an audit or designing a programme in a healthcare organisation. Some assessment points have two elements, indicated (a) and (b). A separate response should be entered in the checklist for both. Other systems for review of audit projects or programmes are discussed in *Stage Five: sustaining improvement.*

Audit projects

Number	Assessment point	Key point/key note	Yes	No	No information
A	**Topics**				
1	The reason for selecting the topic is clear and appropriate.	Clinical audit is used to improve aspects of care over a wide variety of topics. It is also used in association with changes in systems of care, or to confirm that current practice meets the expected levels of performance.	☐	☐	☐
2	Staff are enabled to suggest topics for audit.	The participation of staff in selecting topics enables concerns about care to be reported and addressed. Participation in choice of topic is not always necessary, but may have a role in reducing resistance to change.	☐	☐	☐
B	**Criteria and levels of performance**				
3	Explicit criteria are used.	Explicit rather than implicit criteria should be preferred.	☐	☐	☐
4	The criteria (a) relate to important aspects of care, and (b) are measurable.	Criteria should relate to important aspects of care and be measurable.	☐	☐	☐
5	The criteria are justified by relevant research evidence or guidelines.	Systematic methods should be used to derive criteria from evidence. These include methods for deriving criteria from good-quality guidelines or from reviews of the evidence.	☐	☐	☐
6	Explicit methods are used where criteria are selected by consensus.	If criteria incorporate, or are based on, the views of professionals or other groups, formal consensus methods are preferable.	☐	☐	☐

Number	Assessment point	Key point/key note	Yes	No	No information
7	If standards are specified, they are based on levels of performance reported by others or derived through the use of benchmarking.	There is insufficient evidence to determine whether it is necessary to set target levels of performance in audit. However, reference to levels achieved in audits undertaken by other professionals is useful.	☐	☐	☐
8	Benchmarks are used, if necessary, to set appropriate target levels of performance.	In some audits, benchmarking techniques could help participants in audit to avoid setting unnecessarily low or unrealistically high target levels of performance.	☐	☐	☐
9	The choice of type of criteria is appropriate to the topic and objectives of the audit.	Clinical audit can include assessment of the process and/or outcome of care. The choice depends on the topic and the objectives of the audit.	☐	☐	☐
10	Where the criteria relate to the process of care, evidence is available to confirm that process influences outcome.	Provided that research evidence confirms that clinical care processes have an influence on outcome, measurement of the process of care is generally more sensitive and provides a direct measure of the quality of care.	☐	☐	☐
11	Where outcomes are assessed in the audit, they can be related to the process of care.	Measurement of outcome can be used to identify problems in care, provided the outcomes are clear, influenced by process, and occur within a short period.	☐	☐	☐
12	In comparative audits of outcome, case mix adjustment is performed.	Adjustment for case mix is generally required for comparing the outcomes of different providers.	☐	☐	☐

continued

Number	Assessment point	Key point/key note	Yes	No	No information
C	**Data sources and collection**				
13	Ethical issues are identified and addressed appropriately.	Health service professionals must be aware of the ethical implications of and their responsibilities under the Data Protection Act (1998) when collecting data and presenting results.	☐	☐	☐
14	The parameters of the audit are specified.	Every audit should define the patients to be included, the aspects of care under review, and the time period over which the criteria apply.	☐	☐	☐
15	Appropriate samples are used where sampling is necessary.	Health service professionals need to be able to apply appropriate sampling techniques.	☐	☐	☐
16	The method used to identify patients for inclusion has been tested for completeness, or more than one method is used.	Patient registers are used to identify patients, but registers can be incomplete. The identification of patients using several sources can be an appropriate response.	☐	☐	☐
17	Where records are used as the source of data, their completeness has been assessed or more than one source of data is used.	Although clinical records are frequently used as the source of data, they are often incomplete. The collection of data from several sources can help to overcome this problem.	☐	☐	☐
18	Relevant routinely available data are used if available.	If routinely collected data are available, they may be appropriate for use in clinical audit.	☐	☐	☐

Number	Assessment point	Key point/key note	Yes	No	No information
19	Steps are taken to ensure the consistency of data extraction from records: for example, training of data extractors and use of specifically developed data forms.	When collecting data, a carefully developed data abstraction tool is recommended. Training data abstractors can improve data consistency.	☐	☐	☐
D	**Changing performance**				
20	The barriers to change are investigated prior to planning implementation.	An investigation of potential barriers to change assists in the development of implementation plans.	☐	☐	☐
21	Appropriate methods are used to identify barriers to change.	Teams undertaking audit that are appropriately supported and able to use a variety of techniques can identify potential barriers and develop practical implementation plans.	☐	☐	☐
22	The implementation plan takes the identified barriers into account in selecting methods to change performance.	A systematic approach to implementation appears to be more effective. Such an approach includes the identification of local barriers to change, the support of teamwork, and the use of a variety of specific methods.	☐	☐	☐
23	In planning change, contextual factors are taken into account.	Contextual factors influence the likelihood of change. These include the significance of change to service users, the effectiveness of teamwork, and the organisational environment.	☐	☐	☐
24	Methods additional to feedback are used to implement change.	Those planning audits should avoid relying on feedback alone as the method of implementing change; although feedback of data alone can occasionally be effective, change is much more likely if it forms part of a more complex set of change processes/interventions.	☐	☐	☐

continued

Number	Assessment point	Key point/key note	Yes	No	No information
25	Educational materials such as guidelines are not used as the sole method of implementing change.	The dissemination of educational materials, such as guidelines, has little effect unless accompanied by the use of selected implementation methods.	☐	☐	☐
26	Methods demonstrated as more likely to be effective are used, for example interactive education, reminders, or system changes.	Interactive educational interventions including outreach, service user and/or professional reminders (whether manual or computerised), decision support, and system change can sometimes, but not always, be effective.	☐	☐	☐
27	The implementation plan includes the use of more than one method.	In audit, the use of multifaceted interventions chosen to suit the particular circumstances is more likely to be effective in changing performance than the use of a single intervention alone.	☐	☐	☐
E Service users					
28	Users are consulted about the choice of (a) topic and (b) criteria.	The priorities of those receiving care can differ quite markedly from those of clinicians. Service users should therefore be involved in the clinical audit process.	☐	☐	☐
29	Methods are used to include users at each stage of the audit.	There are practical approaches for user involvement in all stages of audit, including the design, the collection of data about performance, and in implementing change.	☐	☐	☐

Audit programmes

Number	Assessment point	Key point/key note	Yes	No	No information
30	There is an identifiable audit programme with clear leadership	Clinical audit projects are best conducted within a structured programme, with effective leadership, participation by all staff, and an emphasis on team working and support.	☐	☐	☐
31	The audit programme is integrated into the organisation's management and planning systems.	Improvement in care implemented as a part of clinical audit must be monitored, evaluated, sustained, and reinforced within a supportive environment.	☐	☐	☐
32	The clinical audit programme is explicitly integrated with clinical governance.	Clinical governance programmes offer a structure to support efforts to make improvements, including personal professional development, support of teams, and clear accountability.	☐	☐	☐
33	The organisation involves the clinical audit programme in the development of strategies for change.	Structures and systems must be developed to enable organisations to integrate improvements within a planned strategy.	☐	☐	☐
34	The audit programme has policies and methods for actively developing the desired culture.	A culture is required that makes the user's experience the primary motivation for improvements, creates confident staff who do not fear reporting or confronting inadequate performance, and has clear and constant objectives.	☐	☐	☐

continued

Number	Assessment point	Key point/key note	Yes	No	No information
35	The audit programme includes systems to monitor structured improvements.	Systems, structures, and specific mechanisms are available for monitoring sustained improvement.	☐	☐	☐
36	Participation of all health professionals is actively promoted by explicit methods.	Those involved in organising clinical audit programmes must consider various methods of engaging the full participation of all health service staff.	☐	☐	☐
37	The audit programme encourages the participation of staff in selecting topics.	The participation of staff in selecting topics enables concerns in care to be reported and addressed. Participation in choice of topic is not always necessary, but may have a role in reducing resistance to change.	☐	☐	☐
38	Teams undertaking audit are supported by their organisations, including the provision of training in (a) identifying barriers and (b) planning implementation.	Teams undertaking audit that are appropriately supported and able to use a variety of techniques can identify potential barriers and develop practical implementation plans.	☐	☐	☐
39	The organisation takes note of the needs of audit when developing information technology systems.	Electronic information systems can contribute to audit in many ways, including: improving access to research evidence; identifying users; collecting data; prompting change through record templates; and enabling revised systems of care to be introduced.	☐	☐	☐
40	The organisation provides protected time for audit.	The most frequently cited barrier to successful audit is the failure of organisations to provide sufficient protected time for healthcare teams.	☐	☐	☐

Number	Assessment point	Key point/key note	Yes	No	No information
41	The organisation arranges for the provision of training in the skills of clinical audit.	Organisations should ensure that their healthcare staff learn the skills of clinical audit.	☐	☐	☐
42	The organisation provides adequate funds for audit.	Organisations must recognise that clinical audit requires appropriate funding.	☐	☐	☐
43	The organisation has arrangements for responding to the cost implications of the findings of audits.	Organisations need to recognise that improvements in care resulting from clinical audit can increase costs.	☐	☐	☐
44	Alternative models of audit such as delay pattern analysis or critical incident review may form part of the audit programme, but they are used to supplement and not replace traditional audit incorporating the audit cycle.	Alternative models of monitoring healthcare provision, such as delay pattern analysis and critical incident review, can assist with identifying and investigating certain deficiencies in care. The most effective approaches for ensuring that these methods lead to improved care are uncertain.	☐	☐	☐
45	The organisation assesses the quality of audit.	Organisations can use recognised assessment techniques to evaluate the quality of audit carried out by healthcare professionals.	☐	☐	☐

Appendix VII: approach to examining clinical audit during a clinical governance review used by the Commission for Health Improvement

When conducting a clinical governance review of an NHS organisation, CHI examines the following **clinical governance themes** (*see* Table A) across a number of **review issues** (*see* Table B for the specific review issues for clinical audit).

Table A. Clinical governance themes

Theme	Examples of issues that are covered by each theme
Accountabilities and structures	• Clarity and effectiveness of committee responsibilities • Clarity and effectiveness of staff responsibilities at all levels in the organisation (Board; top management team; directorate teams) • Adequacy of monitoring and reporting arrangements
Strategies and plans	• Extent to which there is a coherent strategy for the activity . . . • . . . that is broken down into actionable plans and is resourced (staff, budget) • Extent to which strategies and plans for different clinical governance activities are connected to wider quality improvement programmes • Involvement in the development of strategies and plans of: – patients and the public – health economy partners • Resources (staff and budget) to support the implementation of the strategy

continued

Table A. (*continued*)

Theme	Examples of issues that are covered by each theme
Application of policies, strategies and plans	• Extent to which systems are implemented and operational • Effectiveness of communication to staff, and their understanding, of their responsibilities • Extent of: – staff involvement in the activity – multi-disciplinary involvement – team-based involvement – cross-team involvement – cross-organisation involvement
Quality improvements and learning	• Extent to which information from the activity is considered systematically • Extent to which use of the information has lead to quality improvements • Dissemination of lessons learnt and whether far organisation-wide improvements have resulted
Resources and training for staff and patients	• Access to, and use of, resources to support essential processes and systems, e.g. – information and means of accessing it – human and financial resources to support systems • Uptake of training by staff

Table B. Review issues for clinical audit

	Accountabilities and structures
1	Committee structure for clinical audit
2	Staff responsibilities for clinical audit
3	Reporting and monitoring – to/by management teams, committees and the board
	Strategies and plans
4	Strategy for clinical audit – including priority given to participation in national, regional and local audits – and programmes
5	Integration of clinical audit with quality improvement programmes, e.g. to audit compliance with evidence-based practice protocols, guidelines and care pathways etc
6	Involvement of patient/service users and carers in clinical audit strategy and programme development
7	Involvement of partners in cross-organisational clinical audit
8	Support and resources for clinical audit including: • central clinical audit unit to support audit design, data collection and analysis • budgets for clinical audits

continued

	Application of policies, strategies and plans
9	Clinical audits carried out including: • connections with other clinical governance activities • staff awareness and involvement
10	Participation in national confidential enquiries
	Quality improvements and learning
11	Processes to consider the results of clinical audits
12	Compliance with evidence-based practice shown by audits
13	Quality improvements as a result of clinical audits
14	Dissemination of lessons learnt from clinical audit
	Resources and training for staff
15	Training and development for staff in audit skills

Appendix VIII: recommendations from the *Report of the Public Inquiry into Children's Heart Surgery at the Bristol Royal Infirmary 1984–1995* (2001) and the Government's response (2002)

Competent healthcare professionals

Broadening the notion of professional competence

57 Greater priority than at present should be given to non-clinical aspects of care in six key areas in the education, training and continuing professional development of healthcare professionals:

- skills in communicating with patients and with colleagues
- education about the principles and organisation of the NHS, and about how care is managed, and the skills required for management
- the development of teamwork
- shared learning across professional boundaries
- clinical audit and reflective practice
- leadership.

We agree. We are working with regulatory and professional bodies and educators to ensure that from 2002 these core skills are included in all NHS funded professional programmes and clinical undergraduate training.

Care of an appropriate standard

Standards of care: NHS organisations

130 There must be a single, coherent, coordinated set of generic standards: that is, standards relating to the patient's experience and the systems for ensuring that care is safe and of good quality (for example corporate management, clinical governance, risk management, clinical audit, the management and support of staff, and the management of resources). Trusts must comply with these standards.

We agree. Clinical governance already provides a comprehensive framework against which trusts' services can be judged. In addition, all trusts are required by the Treasury to maintain effective systems of financial, organisational and clinical controls.

Monitoring standards and performance

Local monitoring

143 The process of clinical audit, which is now widely practised within trusts, should be at the core of a system of local monitoring of performance. Clinical audit should be multidisciplinary.

We agree. Multi-disciplinary clinical audit is already a key feature of clinical governance.

144 Clinical audit must be fully supported by trusts. They should ensure that healthcare professionals have access to the necessary time, facilities, advice, and expertise in order to conduct audit effectively. All trusts should have a central clinical audit office which coordinates audit activity, provides advice and support for the audit process, and brings together the results of audit for the trust as a whole.

We agree in principle. Each trust has a lead individual with responsibility for clinical audit and all doctors are required to participate in clinical audit programmes. It is for individual trusts to decide how clinical audit activity should be supported locally, as part of clinical governance.

145 Clinical audit should be compulsory for all healthcare professionals providing clinical care and the requirement to participate in it should be included as part of the contract of employment.

We agree. This is already being addressed for doctors through the introduction of appraisal as a contractual requirement and the impending introduction of FMC revalidation. Trusts are responsible for providing the time and resources to enable multi-disciplinary audit to take place.

National monitoring

146 The monitoring of clinical performance at a national level should be brought together and coordinated in one body: an independent Office for Information on Healthcare Performance. This Office should be part of CHI.

We agree. Proposals for an independent new Office for Information on Health Care Performance within CHI are included in the NHS and Health Care Professions Bill. Though the detailed remit and functions of the Office have yet to be finalised, the Office will collect, analyse and publish reports on clinical and other NHS data. The Office will also develop a clinical audit programme (to include audits currently within the NICE work programme).

147 The Office for Information on Healthcare Performance should supplant the current fragmentation of approach through a programme of activities involving the coordination of the various national audits. In addition to its other responsibilities, the new system should provide a mechanism for surveillance whereby patterns of performance in the NHS which may warrant further scrutiny can be identified as early as possible.

We agree. The Office for Information on Health Care Performance should undertake this task. The assessment, commissioning and surveillance of clinical audit systems will be key functions of the Office.

Information systems

148 The current 'dual' system of collecting data in the NHS in separate administrative and multiple clinical systems is wasteful and anachronistic. A single approach to collecting data should be adopted, which clinicians can trust and use and from which information about both clinical and administrative performance can be derived.

We agree. Those responsible for the separate administration and clinical audit databases are already working together to develop an approach which will avoid duplication. Implementation of Information for Health *will provide the basis for a single approach to collecting data for both clinical and administrative needs through the electronic patient record, which will be introduced by 2005.*

149 Steps should be taken nationally and locally to build the confidence of clinicians in the data recorded in the Patient Administration Systems in trusts (which is subsequently aggregated nationally to form the Hospital Episode Statistics). Such steps should include the establishment by trusts of closer working arrangements between clinicians and clinical coding staff.

150 The Hospital Episode Statistics database should be supported as a major national resource which can be used reliably, with care, to undertake the monitoring of a range of healthcare outcomes.

We agree. A number of steps have been taken to engage clinicians with the value of the data recorded in the Patient Administration System and Hospital Episode Statistics. These include a major consultation on performance indicators, discussions with the BMA about how HES data can be used to monitor clinical quality and research into how HES can be used on a routine basis to identify areas of possible clinical concern.

We recognise the importance of HES as the key database to underpin the whole of the clinical governance programme for the foreseeable future. Our investment includes work on a new contract and tendering the service for supplying HES data. This will deliver improvements in service and create the opportunity to extend the scope of HES to include outpatient and accident and emergency data, and data from the private sector. We are working to make the HES data more accessible to those in the service and to link it with ONS mortality data to provide a more effective measured clinical outcome.

151 Systems for clinical audit and for monitoring performance rely on accurate and complete data. Competent staff, trained in clinical coding and supported in their work, are required: the status, training, and professional qualifications of clinical coding staff should be improved.

We agree. A re-evaluation of the training infrastructure for clinical coders will commence in 2002. The results of this evaluation will lead to a range of measures to improve the training and career structure of clinical coders. These measures will begin to come on stream in 2003.

152 The system of incentives and penalties to encourage trusts to provide complete and validated data of a high quality to the national database should be reviewed. Any new system must include reports of each trust's performance in terms of the quality and timeliness of the submission of data. The systems within a trust for producing data of a high quality, and its performance in returning such data in a timely manner to the national database, should be taken into account in the process of validating and revalidating the trust.

We agree. For the first time, we will include a data quality indicator in the annual NHS Performance Indicators. CHI has also been looking at the quality of data available to trusts in its regular reviews of clinical governance. In addition, the NHS Information Authority has been commissioned to develop a data quality strategy to support the NHS modernisation agenda by September 2002. This strategy will cover roles and responsibilities at all levels, training needs, making data quality an integral part of all data sets and collection initiatives and the feedback of data as a key driver to data quality.

153 At national level, the indicators of performance should be comprehensible to the public as well as to healthcare professionals. They should be fewer and of high quality, rather than numerous but of questionable or variable quality.

We agree. We have recently undertaken a wide ranging consultation with the NHS and public on which performance indicators should be published. In September 2001, we published six high-level indicators against which acute trusts were 'star' rated.

154 The need to invest in world-class IT systems must be recognised so that the fundamental principles of data collection, validation and management can be observed: that data be collected only once; that the data be part and parcel of systems used to support healthcare professionals in their care of patients; and that trusts and teams of healthcare professionals receive feedback when data on their services are aggregated.

We agree. We are investing in the Information for Health *strategy. Electronic patient records will be available by 2005.*

Publication of information about performance and standards

155 Patients and the public must be able to obtain information as to the relative performance of the trust and the services and consultant units within the trust.

We agree. Performance indicators for each trust will be published soon. Further development work is needed before information can be published on services and particular specialties. The Office for Information on Health Care Performance will publish independent information on NHS performance. We wrote, with the support of the BMA, to NHS consultants in December 2001 telling them of our intentions to use available data to publish performance information at consultant team level. We will work with the medical profession to improve local data collection.

156 As part of their Annual Reports trust boards should be required to report on the extent of their compliance with national clinical standards. These reports should be made public and be made available to CHI.

We agree. Trusts are already required annually to produce clinical governance reports and to report progress in implementing NSFs and NICE guidelines. These reports are both public and available to CHI.

Appendix IX: lessons learnt from the National Sentinel Audit Programme

The National Institute for Clinical Excellence (NICE) inherited a programme of national audits projects commissioned by the Department of Health. Ten of these projects, termed National Sentinel Audits (NSA), were commissioned at the same time towards the end of 1997 (*see* Appendix III).

National audit projects must add value to the NHS and facilitate improvements in patient care. It is important that the lessons learnt from these projects influence the design and management of future projects. Knowledge of the successful aspects of these projects as well as the lessons learnt will inform the commissioning and managing of future national audit projects.

Feedback from a wide range of sources has contributed to this Appendix, including that from:

- clinical audit staff at a number of conference sessions including *Clinical Audit '98* and *Clinical Excellence 2000*
- NSA project leads and regional audit staff at a meeting hosted by the National Centre for Clinical Audit in February 1999
- delegates at a national audit workshop hosted by NICE in March 2000
- a review of all the completed national audit projects
- project leads of national audit projects
- centres that work with the Institute on clinical audit, including the National Collaborating Centres
- local NHS staff that have taken part in national audit projects.

Successes

The sentinel audit programme has demonstrated how audit can constructively assist NHS clinical and non-clinical staff to work together towards delivering improved patient care. Some national audit projects have been associated with significant improvements in the quality of care provided in a number of NHS services (e.g. stroke care).

Positive attributes of sentinel audit projects included:

- developing flagship methodologies
- clarifying national standards
- raising the profile of clinical audit
- encouraging a shared enthusiasm for the constructive use of clinical audit
- raising the profile of specific clinical topics
- facilitating national and local comparison of quality of care
- facilitating the opportunity for clinical benchmarking.

Lessons learnt

The lessons learnt from the national sentinel audit programme can be divided into two broad categories:

- project management, including topic selection, planning and resources, and communication
- project methodology, including design, data issues, implementability, stakeholder involvement, and the provision of support for local improvement.

Project management

Topic selection

Lesson 1: The method for gathering and prioritising topics for national comparative audit should be as transparent as possible and involve service providers, users and NHS staff.

National Sentinel Audit topics chosen were of varying relevance and interest to the service. They did not always match local priorities or national policy objectives.

Planning and resources

Lesson 2: Detailed information should be provided as early as possible and again at the recruitment stage to facilitate planning for participation in the project.

The expectation for improvements in patient care should be explicitly articulated in the recruitment documents to engage the enthusiasm of local staff. Advance notices and recruitment documents should make available the project objectives, an outline of the proposed audit protocol, proposed networking opportunities, and plans for supporting local improvement initiatives.

Lesson 3: Adequate time is required for the project leads to engage relevant staff within NHS organisations, and for the organisation to plan their involvement in the project.

Early distribution of the audit protocol including details of the cost of participation, estimated number of cases to be audited, and the time required to audit an average set of case notes would facilitate local planning for the resources required to participate (e.g. budgeting for recruitment of data collection/entry staff, cost of notes retrieval etc.).

Lesson 4: National audit projects are resource intensive at both national and local level. Projects will require a significant commitment from local NHS organisations. Start dates within a programme of national audits should take account of local business planning cycles and be staggered to assist capacity management within the NHS.

Scheduling and planning issues were identified within the NSA programme. Many of the projects were started at the same time, leading to capacity problems in the NHS at key stages (e.g. during data collection). From the perspective of the project leads, these problems arose from the tight time frame of the bidding and funding mechanism.

Communication

Lesson 5: Communication should take place via agreed communication channels such as professional networks and via clinical governance leads in NHS organisations.

From the perspective of NHS staff, recruitment of NHS organisations was carried out through many uncoordinated channels. Project leads spread the recruitment net wide via professional networks, as endorsement by the relevant professional bodies is very important. However there was little direct communication with clinical audit departments. Although local 'sign up', leadership and internal communication are primarily local issues, there is a need to understand the role of staff responsible for project and change management locally and the important part they can play in these projects.

Lesson 6: Stakeholders should be kept well informed. Clear, effective, two-way communication channels should be established with the NHS organisations including those that are not yet able to participate in order to maximise the impact of the audit on improving patient care.

Newsletters, conference and journal communications, e-mail lists, and project websites are ways of keeping all stakeholders up to date with progress and forthcoming events.

Lesson 7: Networking opportunities are valued by practitioners and should be made available at national, regional, and local level.

Workshops are reported to have enabled the development of supportive relationships between participants. Regional opportunities were particularly appreciated, as this minimised time spent away from the workplace and created a sense of local solidarity. Such multidisciplinary meetings allowed discussion of the implications of local results within the national audit.

There are particular logistical challenges of communicating with numerous primary healthcare teams in England and Wales and encouraging them to take part in national audit projects. The need to support primary care teams, and the variety of data recording systems that are in operation should be appreciated.

Project methodology

Design

Lesson 8: The design of a national audit project should conform to the current best practice principles for a clinical audit project and ensure that change is implemented.

National projects that do not audit practice against agreed criteria should be referred to as a baseline survey. Without adherence to principles of best practice in clinical audit at a national level, local initiatives to enthuse clinicians about the benefits of participating in clinical audit (i.e. change and improvement) are seriously undermined.

Some of the national sentinel audits were surveys in clinical areas where no commonly agreed standards of care existed.

Lesson 9: Adequate time should be spent ensuring that the design of the national audit project is right. Poor design can result in an audit that doesn't benefit patients or staff and can be wasteful of time and resources. It should be possible to judge from the audit protocol whether the proposed audit will enable care to be reliably assessed against the criteria.

Considerable effort is required to develop a data collection tool that is unambiguous and reliable. Stakeholders and audit specialists working in the NHS should be involved from the outset to refine the design.

Lesson 10: The design of the audit tool should be kept as straightforward as possible and the amount of data to be collected kept to a minimum.

Collecting more data than is absolutely necessary creates more work for staff and increases the chance that data will be collected hastily or inaccurately. In the presence of good quality baseline data the number of variables for which data are collected should be reduced to the minimum. Piloting should be used to establish the minimum dataset required to permit statistically robust conclusions to be drawn.

Lesson 11: The methodology for data validation and analysis should be transparent. Transparency raises the credibility of data compared at national level and highlights local data quality issues.

Centres leading national audit projects should share knowledge of methodological approaches to data entry and analysis. Common processes should allow errors in data entry or analysis to be identified and rectified quickly to ensure ongoing confidence in the results returned to the NHS.

Lesson 12: The commissioning of a national audit tool should be accompanied by a package of resources including supportive information on setting up the audit, sample size, how to involve service users, and how to interpret and take action on the results. The data collection tool should be supported by, and cross-referenced to, suitable educational material.

The purpose of audit is to bring about improvements in care. Local NHS staff appreciated support in addressing changes required as a result of audit.

Implementability

Lesson 13: The audit tool should be subjected to robust formal piloting using a randomly selected group of clinicians and audit staff working in the NHS, avoiding the bias associated with self-selected groups of enthusiasts.

In one national audit tool, questions were considered unclear and practitioners were left feeling that their views on how to improve the data collection tool had not been heard. Practitioners felt that the tool had been developed by experts with no feel for the 'real world'.

Lesson 14: All national audits should have a clear data collection strategy. The data entry and analysis framework should be appropriately designed for the clinical setting in which the audit is being conducted.

Areas not supported by adequate IT may require central analysis of the data or the provision of a simple analysis tool for use locally. One national audit provided clear guidance on how and when to collect the data, how to fill in the forms, and couriers were sent to collect data from hospitals at set times. Analysis of results was provided within weeks. The level of IT support needed from local IT departments and via a project helpdesk facility has been considerable during current national comparative audit projects.

Stakeholder involvement

Lesson 15: All groups with an interest in the aspects of care covered by the proposed national audit project should be involved.

Stakeholders should be consulted on the scope, design, and presentation of the results and where appropriate should be actively involved in developing the review criteria and establishing action plans for change.

Support for improvement

Lesson 16: Mechanisms to maximise organisational support and commitment should be invoked at the recruitment stage. Projects should be embedded into clinical governance strategies. Successful methods for supporting change should be shared.

> In sites where there was visible management support and commitment, both in terms of time and resources, respondents were clear that the national audit project had been successful. However, where such support and commitment was seen to be absent, a number of difficulties were experienced.

Lesson 17: Statistically robust results presented to the NHS in an easily understandable format and within a reasonable time frame can provide a powerful driver for change locally.

> Timely reporting of the results is crucial, otherwise the relevance of data collected lessens and there may be reduced interest in the report.

Lesson 18: Results should be presented to allow organisations to see clearly whether they are achieving the expected best practice, and to compare their performance against similar health economies.

> Within some of the national audit projects the comparisons to 'what is possible' in other units through benchmarking added value to the results and facilitated change.

Appendix X: list of desirable characteristics of review criteria

The characteristics are ranked in order of importance as rated by an expert panel (the most highly rated characteristic is first, and the lowest rated last)

From Hearnshaw HM, Harker RM, Cheater FM, Baker RH, Grimshaw GM. Expert consensus on the desirable characteristics of review criteria for the improvement of healthcare quality. *Quality in Health Care* 2001; **10**: 173–8.

- Criteria are described in unambiguous terms
- Criteria are based on a systematic review of research evidence
- The validity of identified research is rigorously appraised
- Criteria include clear definitions of the variables to be measured
- Criteria explicitly state the patient populations to which they apply
- Criteria are capable of differentiating between appropriate and inappropriate care
- Criteria are linked to improving health outcomes for the care being reviewed
- Criteria explicitly state the clinical settings to which they apply
- The collection of information required for criteria-based review minimises demands on staff
- The method of selecting criteria is described in enough detail to be repeated
- Criteria are accompanied by clear instructions for their use in reviewing care
- The systematic review used to guide the selection of criteria is up to date
- Criteria are pilot tested for practical feasibility
- Criteria include aspects of care that are relevant to patients
- The collection of information for criteria-based review is acceptable to those patients whose care is being reviewed
- The bibliographic sources used to identify research evidence are specified
- In selecting criteria, decisions on trade-offs between outcomes from different treatment options are stated
- The collection of information required for criteria-based review minimises demands on patients
- The method of synthesising evidence and expert opinion is made explicit

- Criteria are prioritised according to the quality of supporting evidence
- Criteria are prioritised according to their impact on health outcomes
- The criteria used to assess the validity of research are stated
- Similar criteria should emerge if other groups review the same evidence
- The collection of information for criteria-based review is acceptable to those staff whose care is being reviewed
- Expert opinion is included in the process of developing review criteria
- Criteria used in previous quality reviews of the same clinical topic are considered for inclusion

Appendix XI: review of the evidence

Authors

Richard Baker, Keith Stevenson, Elizabeth Shaw, and Sarah Redsell
Clinical Governance Research & Development Unit, Department of General Practice & Primary Health Care, University of Leicester
Clare Morrell and Ross Scrivener
Royal College of Nursing

Acknowledgements

We thank the peer reviewers who provided helpful comments on various drafts of the review: Alan Breen, Francine Cheater, Yvonne Doyle, Nancy Dixon, Debra Humphris, Peter Littlejohns, David Murray and Elizabeth Davies.

The preparation of the review was funded by the National Institute for Clinical Excellence.

Contents

Preface 134
1 Introduction 134
2 Methods used in audit 136
3 The organisation of audit 149
4 Reviews of methods of implementing change 154
5 Discussion and conclusions 163
6 References 165
Annex 1 190

Preface

This review summarises literature about clinical audit, its effectiveness, methods of undertaking audit, and how audit projects and programmes are most appropriately coordinated and run. The evidence was used to underpin *Principles for Best Practice in Clinical Audit* – and the key points that emerged from the evidence can be found in Appendix V.[1] The review is intended for staff in the NHS with particular interest in, or responsibility for, clinical audit and clinical governance. It builds on previous reviews and provides guidance on aspects of audit and reference to relevant publications. It does not give guidance on how to undertake or manage audit, and readers should, in the first instance, consult *Principles for Best Practice in Clinical Audit*.

1 Introduction

Clinical audit is a quality improvement process that seeks to improve patient care and outcomes through systematic review of care against explicit criteria and the implementation of change. Aspects of the structure, processes, and outcomes of care are selected and systematically evaluated against explicit criteria. Where indicated, changes are implemented at an individual, team, or service level and further monitoring is used to confirm improvement in healthcare delivery.

Background

This review updates the 1996 review of the National Centre for Clinical Audit[2] (NCCA) and builds on the 1999 review of systematic reviews of implementation methods undertaken by the Centre for Reviews and Dissemination.[3] The aim of the new review is to identify the key practical, service messages about the conduct of audit in order to underpin *Principles for Best Practice in Clinical Audit*,[1] with the purpose of informing those in the NHS with responsibility for leading or undertaking audit of the most appropriate methods and approaches to adopt.

The principal aim of audit is to improve healthcare, and therefore the new review should consider the effectiveness of audit in promoting improvements. However, in order to make decisions about the best methods to use in different circumstances, information is also needed about how best to undertake the components of audit such as selection of a topic or the development of review criteria. The operation of audit programmes in health service organisations will also influence the extent to which health professionals take part and any ensuing benefits in care, and it follows that information about how audit programmes should be organised is also required. Thus, the review addressed three broad issues:

- the methods to be used in undertaking audit
- the organisation of audit programmes in order to facilitate participation in effective audit
- the effectiveness of audit in implementing change in performance.

These issues are addressed in the following sections. In this first section we outline the background to the review, and in the next section report a review of articles relating to the methods of audit that have been published from 1996. The third section summarises articles published from 1996 concerned with the organisation of audit projects and audit programmes, and in the fourth section we summarise systematic reviews of methods of implementing changes in performance.

The review seeks to identify and summarise relevant articles that provide guidance on the conduct of clinical audit. Staff with a particular interest in or responsibility for leading audit or clinical governance in the NHS should find the review offers practical advice on audit, but it also forms the basis of *Principles for Best Practice in Clinical Audit* that is intended for wider use.[1]

It is important to acknowledge from the outset that we have not undertaken a systematic review. The review did not have a single, focused hypothesis, and included many types of article addressing different aspects of audit. Much of the relevant evidence is in the form of non-experimental studies undertaken in different settings with different designs and concerned with different clinical topics. We have sought to identify and describe the findings in an ordered fashion to promote transparency and enable others to build on the review in the future.

Throughout the review we have included guidance based on the identified articles in the form of key points that are also included in *Principles for Best Practice in Clinical Audit*. The key points highlight aspects indicated as important by the reviewed articles and may be used to summarise best practice in clinical audit. They also form the basis for a checklist (Appendix VI) for use in undertaking or appraising clinical audits. However, it is important to note that the key points are not, nor intended to be, guideline recommendations. They are not based on the level of evidence or formal consensus procedures used in the development of clinical practice guidelines.

The NCCA review

In 1996 the NCCA published *Good Practice in Clinical Audit. A summary of selected literature to support criteria for clinical audit.*[2] The summary of the literature was undertaken to contribute to the development of criteria for good practice in clinical audit, the findings being used together with expert opinion about the essential attributes of audit and the views of health professionals on the conduct of audit in practice. The review was also designed to be a reference for staff with responsibility for the implementation of audit in their healthcare organisations.

The review included (a) an outline of the historical development of the principles of audit dating from the work of Florence Nightingale in the 1850s, (b) a summary of the evidence in relation to each stage in the audit process, and (c) key points about the approaches to use. The review involved searches of relevant bibliographic databases for publications from 1975–1996 supplemented by manual searches. Reports were included if they described key stages of audit, or researched the audit process. Reports of quality improvement activities that were not similar to audit were excluded, as were studies of guideline development or implementation unless the research included audit. The studies identified included reports of tools for the evaluation of audit, reviews of the process of audit, and randomised controlled trials of the effects of audit. The key points that emerged from the articles identified are shown in Annex 1.

The NCCA review considered the evidence in relation to aspects of audit: (a) deciding what, why, and who to audit, (b) defining and measuring current practice, (c) evaluating practice based on measurement, and (d) acting to improve practice and maintaining improvement. In addition, the review drew on the findings of a small number of selected randomised controlled trials pertinent to audit and reviews of audit. The general conclusion was that there was sufficient valid evidence to support the overall efficacy of audit and to identify criteria for good practice. However, the literature was particularly limited with regard to making decisions about what and why to audit, who should be involved, and evaluation prior to acting to improve practice. The findings of the review also identified the need for further research into aspects of audit.

The review and key points provided reliable guidance on the factors influencing the practicality and effectiveness of clinical audit. However, since the report was published in 1996, much new research has been undertaken into audit and quality improvement. Furthermore, there have been changes in health service policy, not least the incorporation of clinical audit into clinical governance, and an up to date review is required.

2 Methods used in audit

Introduction

Audit can be considered to have five principal steps:

- selection of a topic
- specification of appropriate care
- data collection to assess care
- implementation of changes to improve care if necessary
- data collection for a second, or subsequent, time to determine whether care has improved.

The steps have commonly been referred to as the 'audit cycle'. Additional steps may include an analysis of the reasons for current levels of performance prior to selecting strategies to implement change, or three or more data collections to monitor the effects of successive attempts to improve performance.

A variety of methods may be used at each of these stages. Furthermore, in certain types of activity often classified as audit, the traditional stages are not followed. The multiplicity of methods, and the variation in the ways in which they are used, can be confusing. In addition, implementation of change presents a formidable challenge. Therefore, it is not surprising that audits are sometimes poorly executed or fail to bring about desired improvements in care.

The general aim of this review of the methods of audit is to provide practical guidance about the available methods and to highlight those that are most appropriate. The specific elements of audit addressed in the present review were:

1. issues to consider in selecting topics or setting aims
2. methods for developing review criteria and setting levels of performance
3. the role of outcome assessment in audit
4. sources of data for use in audit
5. issues to consider in data collection
6. approaches to use in considering change
7. methods of implementing change
8. the involvement of users (patients, carers, the public) in audit
9. alternative models of collecting data
10. the role of information management and technology (IM&T) in supporting aspects of audit.

Methods of the review

We included all types of study designs, reviews and discussion articles related to audit undertaken by healthcare staff. However, an overview of systematic reviews of methods of implementing change was undertaken separately (*see* Section 4) and therefore randomised trials specifically concerned with methods of implementing change were excluded. We excluded articles not directly concerned with audit, e.g. articles concerned with risk management, clinical governance, performance management etc. We also excluded articles concerned with financial audit, and those reporting studies in which audit was used to refer to data collection from records in the course of evaluations of therapeutic interventions (drugs, surgical procedures). Books about audit or how to conduct audit were also excluded. Articles published before 1996 or not in English were also excluded.

We searched the following bibliographic databases for articles published 1996–2001: Medline, Embase, British Nursing Index, Cinahl, Health Management Information Consortium, PsychINFO, AHMED (Allied and complementary medicine). The search strategies used for Medline are shown in Box 1. The same terms were used in searches of the other databases. The review included all articles relevant to either the methods of audit (any country of origin) or the organisation of audit or audit programmes (from the UK).

We also hand searched the following journals: *Quality in Health Care*, *Bandolier*, *Journal of Clinical Excellence*, *Journal of Clinical Governance/Audit Trends*, *International Journal for Quality in Health Care*, *Journal of Evaluation in Clinical Practice*, and searched the CLIP database.

The bibliographic searches identified 1073 potential articles, and the hand search 328 (1401 in total). Two reviewers independently assessed abstracts of these articles for relevance according to the inclusion and exclusion criteria. We categorised articles according to whether they addressed methods or organisation of audit during review of the abstracts. Copies of the articles were obtained, and 330 articles were included in the review. From those concerned with the methods of undertaking audit, we extracted the following data: country, healthcare setting, year of publication, clinical topics concerned, health professionals involved, design, the methods used, key findings, and principal elements of audit to which the key findings related. The principal elements were categorised as indicated above, and were determined directly from the stated aims of the article, or judged by the reviewers on the basis of each article's conclusions.

Box 1 Search strategies (Medline format)

(a)		Number of articles
1	exp dental audit/ or exp management audit/ or exp medical audit/ or exp nursing audit/ or "audit".mp	6 207
2	Benchmark$.tw	1 035
3	1 or 2	7 062
4	og.xs.	226 021
5	3 and 4	3 635
6	exp evaluation studies/	124 943
7	5 and 6	446
8	limit 7 to (english language and yr = 1996-2001)	316

(b)		Number of articles
1	exp dental audit/ or exp management audit/ or exp medical audit/ or exp nursing audit/	4 796
2	1 or (audit or audits or auditors or auditing or auditor or benchmark$).mp.	7 551
3	exp methods/	8 691
4	2 and (3 or methodolog$.mp.)	250
5	Limit 12 to (english language and yr = 1996–2001)	194

Results

1 Topic/aims

The NCCA review[2] concluded that it appeared desirable that those involved in an audit should participate in selecting the subject and help set objectives using a systematic method. We did not identify studies that compared the consequences of participation or non-participation in selecting the topic of audit. However, in one audit described as external, some health professionals involved did criticise the project and were not convinced by the findings.[4] The topic of this audit was ethnically sensitive practice, and the professionals may have been particularly sensitive to feedback that they perceived as criticism or uncertain about the choice of topic and data collection being undertaken by staff external to the organisation. In contrast, several national monitoring exercises have been undertaken that have included large numbers of professionals even though they did not have the opportunity of taking part in design.[5,6]

Audits were commonly prompted by concerns about problems in care[7,8] although recognition of a problem is not necessarily sufficient to ensure that audit is followed by improved care.[9] Audit may be used in association with the introduction of new systems of care such as policies or protocols in order to evaluate their impact,[10–13] to establish actual practice rather than perceived practice,[14] or to pinpoint high risk aspects of care.[15] For example, Kendall used audit to monitor and evaluate a new system to ensure that patients with myocardial infarcts received thrombolysis.[11]

Audit can provide an overview of service provision[16] or the level of prevalence of a disease in a local geographical area.[17] It may also be used for a wide variety of clinical topics in many different settings,[18–25] but non-clinical topics can also be audited.[26,27]

Key points

- Clinical audit is used to improve aspects of care in a wide variety of topics. It is also used in association with changes in systems of care, or to confirm that current practice meets the expected level of performance.
- The participation of staff in selecting topics enables concerns about care to be reported and addressed. Participation in choice of topic is not always necessary, and may have a role in reducing resistance to change.

2 Development of criteria and levels of performance

In audit, review criteria are generally used for assessing care, and this approach is sometimes referred to as criterion-based audit. The most widely accepted definition of review criteria is that of the Institute of Medicine[28] – 'systematically developed statements that can be used to assess specific healthcare decisions, services, and outcomes'. In contrast, the term 'standard' is used to refer to different concepts. Occasionally it is used as an alternative word for clinical guidelines; it is also used as an alternative to review criteria either with or without a stated target level of performance, and is also used to refer to the observed or desired level of performance. In the interests of clarity we will define standards or target levels of performance as 'the percentage of events that should comply with the criterion'.[29] This is equivalent to the term performance rate, defined as 'a measurement produced by using a performance measure, providing a quantitative evaluation of events related to patient care'.[30]

Criteria

The NCCA report[2] concluded that implicit measures appeared to be less reliable in audit than explicit measures. Whilst this is probably still supported from the articles we reviewed, one of the identified articles argues that in some circumstances, implicit criteria may be more sensitive in identifying particularly important aspects of care.[31] Another study reported the value of an expert panel using their own implicit criteria to rate clinical performance.[32] However, since no direct comparison of implicit and explicit criteria was undertaken, NCCA's preference for explicit criteria should be supported. Corben supports the use of objective criteria in the development of the Buckinghamshire nursing record audit tool.[33]

One article discussed the attributes that review criteria should possess.[34] The principal attribute was that criteria should lead to valid judgements about the quality of care, and therefore criteria should be based on research evidence about the importance of aspects of care.[35,36] Criteria should also relate to aspects of care that are important either to patients or in terms of clinical outcome, and they should be measurable.[37] Several articles considered methods for developing such criteria. Good quality evidence-based guidelines can be used as the starting point for developing criteria.[38–42] Procedures are available for appraising the quality of guidelines,[43] and the examples of development of criteria from guidelines include use of national[38,40,42] and local guidelines[39,44] as the starting point. Since some guideline recommendations may not be directly measurable or not supported by strong evidence of their importance, the number of criteria is generally less than the number of recommendations in the source guideline.[38,41,42] An integrated care pathway may also provide the basis for the development of criteria.[45–48]

A review of relevant literature may also be the basis for criteria, perhaps supplemented by a survey of the views of health professionals.[49] The identification of the care pathway can assist in determining the aspects of care about which evidence is required for the development of criteria.[50]

Consensus methods offer an alternative approach that can be combined with a preliminary literature review[51,52] or used directly.[53–57] A recent review of consensus development methods is available and provides detailed guidance on the most appropriate approaches to use.[58] We did not identify studies comparing the validity of criteria derived from the literature with those developed by consensus, and it should be noted that most methods involved a degree of judgement about which aspects of care are important, even though clear principles for judging importance may be specified.[34,41] Similarly, Shekelle *et al.* have shown that different panels may produce different ratings of appropriateness for the same topic.[59] Criteria development may not always be easy, and Berlowitz *et al.* found that assessment of quality can differ depending on the criteria used.[60] This may result in frustration among those being audited if they recognise the inconsistency.[61]

In developing criteria in local audits, a uni- or multiprofessional group is often given the lead,[49] and some groups used information about local performance to assist in the selection of criteria.[49,62] Local development of criteria requires time and some expertise, but centrally developed sets of criteria are available and have been found to be acceptable in primary care.[63]

Key points

- Explicit rather than implicit criteria should be preferred.
- Systematic methods should be used to derive criteria from evidence. These include methods for deriving criteria from good-quality guidelines or from reviews of evidence.
- Criteria should relate to important aspects of care and be measurable.
- If criteria incorporate, or are based on, the views of professionals or other groups, formal consensus methods are preferable.

Standards/target levels of performance

Relatively few articles reported the use of systematic methods for setting target levels of performance, and the most common approach was informal agreement among the group leading the audit, or among health professionals.[64] In some settings, external standards can be useful.[65] In many audits, no explicit targets are set, and participants merely seek to improve on current performance. In one audit, a matrix was used to scale performance indicators to provide an overall score which was then used as a baseline to measure improvement.[66] We did not find any evidence to suggest that setting target levels of performance increases the likelihood of improvements in performance, and therefore cannot determine whether this is a necessary aspect of audit. However, information about the levels of performance that can be achieved may be helpful when making plans for improvement. Target levels of performance should be examined periodically. As care improves, deviations from criteria may be more likely to be justifiable variation.[67]

Benchmarking

Work has been undertaken in the USA examining systems to derive benchmarks from assessment of the performance of healthcare providers,[68–75] and the use of such methods could help participants in audit set realistic targets or avoid accepting relatively low levels of performance.[76] National audits may provide data for benchmarking.[77] Other authors sought reports of audits undertaken by others to select targets,[40,78,79] or professionals were encouraged to set their own targets.[80]

Key points

- There is insufficient evidence to determine whether it is necessary to set target levels of performance in audit. However, reference to the levels achieved in audits undertaken by other professionals is useful.
- In some audits, benchmarking techniques could help participants in audit to avoid setting unnecessarily low or unrealistically high target levels of performance.

3 Outcomes

In the past, there was a preference for measuring process over outcome, but this view is no longer sustainable. There are arguments for and against the assessment of outcome in audit. The NCCA review identified nine disadvantages to the assessment of outcome alone:[2] outcomes are not a direct measure of performance; adjustment for case mix is required; some outcomes may be delayed; evidence about the impact of some care processes on outcome is limited; not all patients who experience poor process necessarily have a poor outcome; many different factors contribute to eventual outcome; outcomes cannot be improved unless clinicians develop an understanding of how process influences outcome; process measures are less expensive to use; outcome data can be subject to misrepresentation and misunderstanding by the public. Crombie and Davies[83], Marek,[84] and Brook *et al.*[85] in general support these arguments, placing emphasis on the use of measures of processes of care that have been shown by convincing research evidence to influence outcomes.[86] Mant and Hicks also stress the need for careful interpretation of outcome measures.[87]

Nevertheless, other articles present methods of assessing the outcomes of care for some groups of patients.[88–96] The methods used may include patient questionnaires,[97] mortality,[98,99] or symptom scores.[100–102] Other scoring systems have also been described.[103–107] Methods of taking case mix into account have been reported,[98,99,108] but informal accounting for variations in patient populations is often used as an alternative to these formal systems.

The use of outcome assessment is commonest in relation to aspects of care that have clearly defined outcomes that occur within a short period of process. Surgical procedures are an example, and since variations in surgical technique and outcomes have been documented, the routine monitoring of surgical outcomes is clearly justified.[99,100] When there are clear and important measurable outcomes, it can be argued that the assessment of outcomes should be expected. Users' views on the care they have received may also be classified as an outcome, and this is discussed further in relation to user involvement in audit (*see* page 147).

Key points

- Audit can include the assessment of the process and/or outcome of care. The choice depends on the topic and the objectives of the audit.
- Provided that research evidence confirms that clinical care processes have an influence on outcome, measurement of the process of care is generally more sensitive and provides a direct measure of the quality of care.
- Measurement of outcome can be used to identify problems in care, provided outcomes are clear, influenced by process and occur within a short period.
- Adjustment for case mix is generally required for comparing the outcomes of different providers.

4 Data sources

Before data can be collected, the patients whose care is of interest must be identified. Various registers are generally used, but it should not be assumed that they are complete or accurate. Cases may be coded incorrectly.[112] The attention given to maintenance of registers can vary between districts, and some districts may not have relevant registers,[113] but the use of several registers or methods of identifying patients can increase the proportion of cases that are detected.[114]

Although clinical records are frequently used as the source of data in audits, several studies indicate that they are often inadequate. Some aspects of care are more likely to be recorded than others[115,116] and one US study suggested that in some cases, aspects of care classified as necessary were indicated as performed in the records although standardised patients reported that they had not been done.[117] In contrast, aspects of care classified as unnecessary were sometimes not recorded although the standardised patients reported they had been performed. The perceptions of some professionals about care given may differ from information contained in the records,[118] different professional groups may record different information,[119] and direct observation can be more accurate than the data in clinical records.[120] The information obtained at post-mortem may also differ from the conclusions of clinical records.[121] However, audit may be used as a method to improve the quality of record keeping.[122] Encounter or registration sheets completed by the practitioner at the time of consultations may be another strategy for collecting information not routinely or reliably recorded in records.[123] Another strategy to overcome the problem presented by clinical records is the use of multiple sources of information,[124,125] but a compromise between data quality and the costs and practicality of collecting data will often be required.[126]

Routine administrative data can often provide information suitable for audit purposes.[127–129] However, Geraci *et al.*[130] found that discharge summaries were poor measures of complication rates, and suggest that such data should not be used as the primary source for identifying patients. Similarly, automatically collected data can provide information, but a 'hybrid' method using chart review and automatically collected data may be more reliable.[131]

Other sources of data also have deficiencies, for example letters between hospitals and general practitioners do not always contain information about all relevant aspects of care.[132] Adverse incidents as sources of data or for identifying patients for audit are also likely to be incomplete,[133,134] although this problem may eventually be addressed as systems to ensure full reporting are introduced.

Key points

- Patient registers are used to identify patients, but registers can be incomplete. The identification of patients using several sources can be an appropriate response.
- Although clinical records are frequently used as the source of data, they are often incomplete. The collection of data from several sources can help to overcome this problem.

5 Data collection and analysis

Data collection in criterion-based audit is generally undertaken to determine the proportion of cases whose care is in accordance with the criteria, although the use of scoring systems has been reported.[139] Routinely collected data may be used if available, making possible repeated data collections with the minimum of extra effort.[140] Data about prescribing offer an example of this approach.[141,142] Data can also be collected through direct observation,[143] or from questionnaire surveys of staff.[144,145]

Clinical records remain the commonest source of data, and approaches have been developed for ensuring consistency in the abstraction of data. Methods have been described for the development of data abstraction forms[145–148] and a number of standard data collection instruments have been developed.[149,150] Training of data abstractors can improve accuracy.[151] The use of a standard proforma may also assist in the reliability of data collection, leading to effective implementation of changes in care.[152–154] The use of multiple sources of data may also improve the completeness and accuracy of data.[125,155] Statistical process control charts appear to provide informative analyses of data, but there are few examples of their use in audit.[156]

Audit does not necessarily require in-depth statistical knowledge, but when designing an audit, sampling and analysis of the data should be considered.[157,158] Khunti *et al.*[159] describe a simple method of reporting audit results that allows rapid consideration of the level of performance reached.

Data collectors should always be aware of their responsibilities to the Data Protection Act[160] and any locally agreed guidelines.[161]

Key points

- If routinely collected data are available, they may be appropriate for use in audit.
- When collecting data, a carefully developed data abstraction tool is recommended. Training of data abstractors can improve data consistency.

6 Considering change

Change does not always occur in audit and consideration of the reasons for failure may take place after the second data collection.[169,170] However, some authors report taking steps before implementing change that helped them develop appropriate implementation plans. Barriers have been identified to the implementation of guidelines,[171] and the identification of such barriers to change beforehand provides an opportunity to devise informed implementation plans. Preparing and planning for action has been identified as a key factor in the success of an implementation initiative.[172]

A small number of articles did report approaches to identifying potential barriers and the development of plans to overcome them. Both Ruston and Lawes[173] and Smith *et al.*[174] reported an assessment by the team responsible for the audit. Information may be provided by data from the first data collection,[175,176] and audit teams themselves can be supported through the facilitation of networking to enable teams to learn from each other[177] or by effective team leadership.[178] Teams can also benefit from using established techniques for identifying problems and proposing possible beneficial changes to the provision of care, for example fishbone charts.[179] A small, local audit may also identify the reasons for poor performance, for example Beaumont reported an audit in a single practice that highlighted shortage of resources as the reason why local practices did not provide care to people with drug addiction.[180] In response, the local health authority made extra resources available.

Several authors argue that audit and change should be housed within improvement programmes,[181,182] or frameworks.[183,184]

Key points

- An investigation of potential barriers to change assists in the development of implementation plans.
- Teams undertaking audit that are appropriately supported and able to use a variety of techniques can identify potential barriers and develop practical implementation plans.

7 Implementing change

The review identified several audits in which change in care had occurred. Simple methods were occasionally effective, for example feedback about the use of X-rays,[187] peer review,[188] or through the use of a patient-held record.[189] However, a feature of many of the audits was the use of several methods together within the context of an implementation plan.[190–193] For example, Cox *et al.* used a mix of methods, including changes to routine systems supported by facilitated teamwork, to plan change.[194]

Hodgkin *et al.* recommended the use of methods tailored to local circumstances, drawing on marketing techniques and coordinating all local agencies involved in care or able to influence change.[195] The provision of clear data, perhaps using modern information systems,[196] and supported by active teamwork, can be effective.[197] Support from the organisation for teamwork appears helpful,[196,198] and resistance to change among local professionals[199] or in the organisational environment or team[200,201] should be considered. Patients themselves may have preferences for care that make change difficult.[202] Attention to systems of care can also be helpful.[174,203–205]

The role of teamwork is illustrated by articles reporting the use of quality management techniques, including rapid cycle improvement,[206] analysis of systems, and facilitation,[194,207] but teams are likely to require long-term support in order to learn and continue to use these methods effectively. Change is not necessarily maintained long-term, and further data collections or systems to maintain change may be required.[208] One study found that appropriate care was only achieved after several rounds of the audit cycle.[209] For some topics, such as adverse incidents, systems for continuous data collection may be justified.[210]

The significance of teamwork, culture, and resistance to change has led several authors to propose frameworks for planning implementation. These usually include analysis of the barriers to change and use of theories of individual, team or organisational behaviour to select strategies to address the barriers.[211–213] We did not identify experimental evaluations of these frameworks, but since they are complex and involve tailoring implementation methods to local circumstances, randomised trials would present difficulties. Finally, the costs of implementation should not be overlooked,[214] and it is possible that less effective but less costly methods would be appropriate in certain circumstances.

Key points

- A systematic approach to implementation appears to be more effective. Such an approach includes the identification of local barriers to change, the support of teamwork, and the use of a variety of specific methods.
- Contextual factors influence the likelihood of change. These include the significance of the change to service users, the effectiveness of teamwork, and the organisational environment.

8 User involvement

We define 'User' as including patients, carers, or potential users of health services. There is a considerable amount written about the importance of user involvement or partnership in healthcare.[220–223] There are also examples of effective user involvement in clinical audit.[224,225]

There is also evidence that users' priorities can differ from those of healthcare professionals and managers.[52,202] The proposition that users should be involved in all stages of the audit process is clear and the review suggests that there is a growing number of studies to support particular methods of including them in audit which result in success in achieving health gain. Users have been involved effectively in panels to select criteria[54] and prioritise topics for audit.[226]

Of the studies that we reviewed, some assessed methods of user involvement. Two were reviews of the level of user involvement in audit.[227,228] Both reviews argued for more user involvement in audit. Other studies demonstrated that users are being involved increasingly in audit and can make a difference to the quality of care. Parr *et al.* involved users in improving care in an audit to influence uptake of aspirin after myocardial infarction.[229] In other projects, patient-held records were used to involve users in implementing improvements in the care of people with asthma[230] and diabetes.[189]

Studies of audits investigating service needs are particularly well served by involving users and users are reported to help drive change. Several studies reported the advantage of user involvement in assessing the service needs of patients and carers.[231–234] Parents and children were interviewed in two studies,[235] Grimes interviewed people with brain tumours,[236] and Kroese *et al.*, people with learning and communication difficulties,[237] indicating that a wide variety of users may be involved. In an audit of pain control after Caesarian section, mothers provided information on the level of pain control.[238] A system of self-medication was introduced and better pain control achieved, illustrating that user involvement can include several elements and lead to better outcomes. Patients have also been successfully involved in helping assess physician style,[239] and assessment of hospital performance has also benefited from systematic gathering of patient data.[240,241]

It is argued that a change of attitude is still required before user involvement is a reality,[242] although there are signs that it is happening and working.[243] Addressing cultural barriers may offer some opportunity to involve users.[110] Staff require organisational support and training to ensure that initiatives involving users are successful.[244]

Key points

- The priorities of those receiving care can differ quite markedly from those of clinicians. Service users should, therefore, be involved in the clinical audit process.

- There are practical approaches for user involvement or participation in all stages of audit, including the design, the collection of data about performance, and in implementing change.

9 Alternative models of collecting audit data

Some articles report audits that present alternative models or approaches for collecting and interpreting data. Many audits identified in the review involved professionals from different healthcare sectors collecting data that monitored the continuity of care across primary/secondary care boundaries. In some this was the principal feature and these have been referred to as interface audits. An audit that monitors the accuracy and consistency of referral letters and discharge summaries is one example.[248] Burrow and Rimmer reported an audit in which general practitioners and psychiatrists worked together.[249]

There are other approaches that have been referred to as audit, although they do not incorporate the full audit cycle. Delay pattern analysis involves the investigation of new diagnoses to identify delays between the presentation of typical symptoms and reaching the diagnosis.[250] We did not identify articles reporting use of this technique as part of a larger project to reduce diagnostic delays. The detailed review of specific cases or critical incidents is described by Robinson and Drinkwater.[251] In this approach, the discussions of the healthcare team were facilitated in order to ensure openness about deficiencies in care.[252] The full impact of this method has yet to be fully evaluated. Both delay pattern analysis and critical incident analysis may be regarded as forms of data collection, and Redpath *et al.* describe the usefulness of this technique.[253] Rapid-cycle data collection as used by teams in quality improvement is beginning to be adopted.[206,254] This approach may have advantages in promoting change, but experience is still limited and it is not yet possible to determine when it is most effective.

Key point

- Alternative models of assessing healthcare provision, such as delay pattern analysis and critical incident review, can assist with identifying and investigating certain deficiencies in care. The most effective approaches for ensuring that these methods lead to improved care are uncertain.

10 The impact of Information Management and Technology (IM&T)

Although computers have long been used to support data management in audit, they can have a much wider role. Of course, computers can be used to collate data[265] and if adequately maintained, databases can be used on a continuous basis to monitor performance and provide regular feedback.[266–268] Computers are also of central importance in the manipulation of data.[269]

However, there are examples of systems being used to integrate the delivery of care and its assessment. Kalayi *et al.* report an audit in which a new IM&T system with electronic records was used to identify patients for inclusion in the audit.[270] In response to the findings of the first data collection, an automated electronic referral system was introduced to ensure that patients received the appropriate care. Computer based record templates can have a role in implementing changes in performance.[271] In another project, the use of a new system with training being provided by the trust IM&T department led to improvements in hospital discharge communications.[272]

O'Brien reported an evaluation of an electronic knowledge management tool,[273] the WAX active library, for use by general practitioners. The use of the system by general practitioners increased over a six month period and doctors rated it as easy to learn, fast to use and preferable to paper for providing information during consultations.

Key point

- Electronic information systems can contribute to audit in many ways, including: improving access to research evidence; identifying users; collecting data; prompting change through record templates; and enabling revised systems of care to be introduced.

3 The organisation of audit

Introduction

Arrangements to facilitate audit were introduced in the NHS from 1991, including the provision of some resources, the creation of audit committees, and the employment of staff to support audit. Thus, for the past ten years, health service organisations have been responsible for programmes of audit that include structures and policies. Although the methods used to undertake audit will influence any improvements achieved, the operation of audit programmes may also have an impact. The objective of this part of the review is to identify the organisational factors that influence participation in, and the effectiveness of, audit.

In 1993, the Department of Health commissioned the CASPE Research Unit to evaluate the national audit programmes. Their findings were published as case studies of successful clinical audit programmes during the mid-1990s. The key features of success identified by the CASPE reports are that audit programmes are directed at quality improvement, are valued and respected by the stakeholders, cover all services, departments and professions, and produce documented and demonstrable improvements in the quality of healthcare provided.[275]

Some of the published findings from CASPE reports pre-date the inclusion criteria for this review. Therefore, this chapter includes some of the more recent CASPE evaluations as well as the evidence from the other studies identified by the literature review.

Methods of the review

This review is concerned with establishing the organisational features that apply particularly to UK healthcare. Every country will have differences in their healthcare organisational culture and these are likely to have particular effects on the success of audit programmes. Furthermore, different quality improvement methods are favoured in different countries. Therefore, only articles concerned with the organisation of UK-based audit are included in this review to eliminate the difficulty of generalising about organisational features from different healthcare systems.

The search described in Section 2 was used to identify articles concerned with the organisation of audit projects or programmes. Articles were classified into either evaluations of audit programmes or methods of evaluating audit. The inclusion and exclusion criteria and search strategies were as described in Section 2.

Results

1 Evaluations of audit programmes

This review aimed to examine whether there is evidence that some ways of organising audit programmes are better than others. It should be noted that some of the studies were conducted over five years ago, before the introduction of clinical governance. The review produced few evaluations of audit programmes from single studies but some consistent messages emerged. There are some methods of organising audit programmes that are better than others.

Features associated with successful audit

The most important message to emerge from the literature is that health service organisations need to create an environment conducive to conducting audit[276–279] and to develop structured programmes[280–283] that have realistic aims and objectives.[278] Features reported as associated with successful audit programmes are leadership[276] and the attitude of senior management.[284] A non-directive, hands-on approach is considered desirable[277,278] However, in organisations without a dedicated audit team, leadership may need developing within existing management structures.[285]

In practical terms, successful audit requires support staff, strategy groups, and regular discussions.[280,286] Skilled facilitation can help with problem relationships and act as a stimulus to maintain quality activities until the clinical team are able to take full responsibility for the audit process.[286–288] Facilitators' experiences suggest that a 'bottom-up' approach to quality and a 'top-down' approach to action and change are needed.[289] Team working has also been identified as important[290] and this may require facilitation. Increased team working has been identified as a secondary benefit of a successful audit.[291]

A full understanding of how 'ownership' by healthcare professionals contributes to the success of an audit has not been established in the literature. Ownership has been defined as 'meaningful' participation that gives staff a sense of control over the direction of the quality improvement programme. It was regarded as one of the key factors that influenced the successful implementation of the national nursing quality programmes.[289] A balance between local involvement and regional standardisation may also contribute to the success of audit.[292]

However, it remains to be established whether ownership should be regarded as an attitude of staff towards the importance and function of audit, or whether it should be seen as a process describing participation. Also, the particular process that leads to acceptance of, and a positive attitude towards audit remains to be fully clarified. Commitment and participation of all staff were considered vital components for successful audit in the CASPE reports[275–278] Two methods of encouraging participation are described in the literature; one involved the setting up of an audit project in which novel approaches were used[293] and the other used the forum of an 'audit club'.[294] Two further studies suggest that involving staff at all stages of the audit cycle is vital to maintain their interest.[295,296]

Walshe and Spurgeon[297] presented a framework for assessing and improving the effectiveness of clinical audit in work commissioned by the NHS Executive in response to recommendations made by the National Audit Office and the Public Accounts Committee in their examination of clinical audit in England. The framework highlights features of effective programmes, including: management and direction, planning, support and resources, coverage and participation, training and skills development, monitoring and reporting, and evaluation (*see* Table 3.6 on CD-ROM).

Particular features of audit programmes (participation, a supportive environment, training and cost) are considered in more detail below.

Key point

- Clinical audit projects are best conducted within a structured programme, with effective leadership, participation by all staff, and an emphasis on team working and support.

Barriers to successful audit

1 Failure to participate and attitudes to audit

There is evidence of variable rates of participation in audit amongst healthcare professionals together with evidence that it has traditionally been dominated by the medical profession.[300–303] Eccles *et al.* suggested that clinical audit remains largely unidisciplinary with few audits initiated collaboratively.[304] Participation in a facilitated programme for primary healthcare teams was reported to be low in one project (6 out of 147 practices)[305] and also in another quality improvement study conducted in primary care.[207] However, others argue that audit is now part of routine practice for nurses.[306]

Participation may be defined in various ways, from taking a peripheral role in an audit at some point in the past two years to initiating and carrying out audits on a regular basis. Therefore, it is difficult to establish the participation rates of doctors, nurses, or allied health professionals. Two studies examined methods of encouraging participation in multidisciplinary audit; one found that involving all stakeholders in the new project was helpful.[293] Another study found that multipractice audits could encourage participation.[307] However, there is insufficient evidence in support of particular methods of encouraging participation, and this is likely to be subject to local variation. It is important to recognise the attitudes of those whose behaviour is being audited, and to modify the audit process to accommodate these views.[308] A relationship has been found between the size of a general practice and participation, suggesting that larger, training practices face fewer obstacles to undertaking audit.[309,310]

In addition to the low levels of participation, failure to continue and complete the audit cycle has been reported,[311–313] which makes it impossible to determine whether the audit has led to any improvements in care.[313]

Key point

- Those involved in organising audit programmes must consider various methods of engaging the full participation of all health service staff.

2 Failure to provide a supportive environment for audit

The organisational environment must be conducive to the development of a successful audit programme.[276–278] Perceived lack of support at all stages, together with a range of structural and organisational problems, are associated with poor progress in conducting audit.[300,316–318] Recent work has pointed to organisational difficulties creating a theory-practice gap for clinicians carrying out audit, one solution being to change the organisational culture to one in which clinical audit is supported and actively encouraged.[319]

The main barrier to audit reported in the literature is a lack of resources,[318] especially time.[319] This includes lack of protected time to investigate the audit topic, collect and analyse data[209,300,317,319] and the time to complete an audit cycle.[311,312]

It follows that audit should be recognised as an important part of clinical practice and those directly involved in audit need to be allocated protected time.

Key points

- Successful clinical audit requires the organisation to promote a culture in which audit is supported and actively encouraged.
- The most frequently cited barrier to successful audit is the failure of organisations to provide sufficient protected time for healthcare teams.

3 Lack of training in audit methodology and evidence-based skills

Health professionals and audit support staff require adequate knowledge and skills for undertaking audit,[275,276] and are keen to learn.[323] Barriers identified in the literature include a lack of training in evidence-based audit skills,[316] and the failure to apply what has already been established.[324] One study found that none of the audits of hypertension included all the criteria considered essential by a panel of experts.[325] In another study, general practitioner trainers were failing to recognise basic audit methodology using a marking schedule they helped to design, a finding that has implications for their ability to teach audit to their registrars and may explain some of the difficulties in implementing audit.[326] Also, there may be confusion between audit as a tool for education and professional development, and audit for monitoring contract performance.[327] Miles *et al.* have suggested that a new training strategy, along with a trial of its effectiveness, is required.[324] A workshop to explore the best ways for health authorities to support best practice has been used to examine the changes which are required.[328]

Key point

- Organisations should ensure that their healthcare staff learn the skills of audit.

4 Cost

There is a limited amount of information about the cost and cost implications of audit. Three small studies identified cost as a barrier to audit although for different reasons. One study considered the cost of data collection,[330] which can be a demanding component of audit.[319] Earnshaw also identified that the costs of conducting audit in one general hospital were high, and recommended that more work be undertaken to determine whether it was cost-effective in improving care.[331] The third study found that applying evidence-based practice significantly increased the cost of treating patients with uncontrolled hypertension.[332] A further study demonstrates the use of a model to estimate the cost utility of clinical audit.[333]

Key points

- Organisations must recognise that audit requires appropriate funding.
- Organisations need to recognise that improvements in care resulting from clinical audit can increase costs.

2 *Methods of evaluating audits*

There is some agreement that evaluating clinical audit programmes is important.[297,334] However, there is no evidence that a particular audit tool is effective in evaluating the quality of clinical audit and the majority have not yet been evaluated for their psychometric properties. On the evidence available, it is not possible to recommend one particular tool.

Walshe and Spurgeon suggest that audit can be evaluated by examining three areas.[297] The first is concerned with the reasons for doing the audit, the second the impact of the audit and the third is the cost. Millard developed a scale to measure the quality of audit projects and found a wide range of responses leading to the conclusion that audit facilitators were not consistent in their responses.[335] Lord and Littlejohns report that a number of different methods have been used to evaluate audit quality,[334] including the development of a tool to assess staff perceptions of the impact of clinical audit,[336] and there is a growing body of evidence regarding good practice that should be utilised by those charged with implementing audit. There are several studies describing methods of evaluating audits,[337–339] and ensuring that audit is central to quality improvement.[340–343] A study commissioned by the Health Technology Assessment programme has developed a tool for assessing methods used to develop review criteria (www.hta.nhsweb.nhs.uk/) (*see* Appendix X).

Key point

- Organisations can use recognised assessment techniques to evaluate the quality of audit carried out by healthcare professionals.

4 Reviews of methods of implementing change

Introduction

During the past decade, interest in methods of improving the performance of health professionals has been intense. In many developed countries, concerns about the quality of care combined with long standing and growing concern about costs have caused policy makers, funders of research programmes, and researchers to seek evidence about the effectiveness of different methods of implementing change. The result has been a steep increase in the number of relevant studies.

Some studies have sought to identify the barriers to improvement, and others have described the experiences of health professionals or teams in implementing change. A number of theoretical frameworks have also been proposed. There have also been a large number of experimental or quasi-experimental studies of various designs, and a growing number of systematic reviews of such studies have been undertaken. Overviews of the many systematic reviews have begun to appear. In this section, we report a summary of systematic reviews, developed from the overview of the NHS Centre for Reviews and Dissemination *Getting Evidence into Practice*.[3] The CRD overview also considered theoretical perspectives on the implementation of change and practical experience, but we have not attempted a review of these issues.

Forty-four systematic reviews were included in the CRD overview. The methods, results, and conclusions of each systematic review were summarised, the reviews being categorised into those involving broad strategies (a variety of interventions targeting a variety of behaviours), reviews of interventions to improve specific behaviours, and reviews of specific interventions. The overview also drew on theoretical perspectives of behaviour change and practical experience.

The general conclusion of the CRD overview from these sources of evidence was that any attempt to change practice should use a systematic approach and involve strategic planning. A diagnostic analysis should be undertaken to inform the design and content of the dissemination and implementation strategies. Various methods may be used to undertake the diagnostic analysis, according to local circumstances, but they may include an assessment of the characteristics of the proposed change that might influence its adoption, assessment of the preparedness to change of the health professionals concerned, and the identification of any external barriers to change. The results of the analysis should be used to inform the design and content of the dissemination and implementation strategies. Broad-based, multifaceted interventions are more likely to be effective, and the extent to which the desired change is achieved should be monitored. Methods may also be needed to maintain change in the long term.

Our particular concern was the effectiveness of audit. In the reviews of interventions to change professional performance, audit is referred to as 'audit and feedback', audit being regarded solely as the collection of data about performance. Feedback is defined by EPOC (Cochrane Effective Practice and Organisation of Care Group) as a summary of clinical performance that may include recommendations for clinical action. It may be in written, electronic, or verbal formats. In audit undertaken in the NHS, a wide variety of implementation methods have been used, and not simply feedback alone. Audit is often used in the NHS, therefore, to indicate a broader range of activities than is defined as audit in the reviews. For clarity, in this section, we use the term 'feedback' rather than 'audit and feedback', and have placed the reviews into three categories: those concerned with the effectiveness of feedback alone, those concerned with the effectiveness of various interventions including feedback, and those reviews concerned with interventions other than feedback.

The general aim of the overview of the reviews was to identify the effectiveness of different methods of implementing change in order to make practical recommendations about the use of methods within the context of audit in the NHS.

Methods

We included systematic reviews of interventions designed to change the performance of health professionals, the outcomes being measures of health professionals' performance and/or healthcare outcomes. We excluded reviews not reporting explicit selection criteria, reviews not reported in English, and overviews of systematic reviews.

Forty-four reviews were identified from the CRD review.[3] To identify recently published reviews, we searched the Cochrane Effective Practice and Organisation of Care Group (EPOC) reviews database, searching for reviews (review as a text word) published from 1999 onwards. This database contains details of articles identified as reviews or meta-analyses of studies relevant to EPOC. We identified 19 reviews that had been published in 1999, and 13 from 2000. There were no reviews identified for 2001. Two reviewers independently assessed these additional 32 reviews to determine their eligibility for inclusion, using the inclusion criteria described above.

Fourteen reviews were excluded, because they either did not report explicit selection criteria or were reviews of a change in service format rather than a change in professional behaviour. The EPOC group listing of Cochrane reviews was also searched and an additional eight reviews were identified. After duplicates were removed, a total of 63 reviews were included in the overview.

Two reviewers independently extracted data from the included reviews about the inclusion criteria, targeted behaviours, implementation methods used, outcome measures reported, and the conclusions. Disagreements between reviewers were resolved through discussion. Data were presented qualitatively to enable broad conclusions to be drawn.

From the reviews of feedback, we sought to determine whether this method could lead to clinically useful improvements in the process and/or outcome of care. From the reviews of audit and feedback and other interventions, we sought to determine the effectiveness of feedback in comparison with other methods, and whether the addition of other methods improves the impact of feedback. From the reviews of interventions other than audit and feedback, we sought to identify effective interventions that could be used in the context of audit in the NHS.

Results of the review

1 Reviews of feedback alone

The objective of this component of the overview was to determine whether this method could lead to clinically useful improvements in the process and/or outcome of care. We identified three reviews that investigated the effect of audit and feedback specifically (*see* Table 4.1 on CD-ROM). In a review of peer-comparison feedback[344] (profiles) in changing practice patterns, 12 trials were identified. Eleven trials had been undertaken in the US, and one in Denmark, the targeted behaviours included prescribing, test ordering, and preventive health screening. There was a statistically significant but modest effect, and the authors of the review were concerned that the costs of providing feedback might outweigh any cost benefits due to changes in care.

The review of Mugford *et al.*[345] was a relatively early example that included 36 studies with historical or concurrent control groups. Feedback that was described as passive – the feedback of statistical information without any discussion or other activity – was reported to be either not effective or of limited effect. More active feedback – preceded by or accompanied with a standard setting exercise or other discussion of practice – was reported as more likely to be effective.

Thomson O'Brien *et al.*[346] included 37 randomised controlled trials. Feedback consisted of different types of information, including summaries of the numbers or costs of diagnostic tests or prescriptions, or compliance scores with review criteria. In some studies, peer-comparison feedback was provided. The frequency of giving feedback varied from once only to repeated feedback at specific intervals. Although most feedback was given in the form of written reports, it was occasionally delivered personally to either individuals or groups of professionals. The review concluded that feedback can be useful, but that the effects are small to moderate. It may be more effective for particular topics such as improvement of prescribing or diagnostic test ordering, but efforts to improve professional performance should not rely solely on this approach.

In these reviews, feedback of information about performance to individuals or groups of professionals is the intervention used to implement change. The reviews concluded that feedback can be effective and clinically useful, but sometimes it is not effective, and even if it is effective, it is only moderately so. In many of the audits undertaken in the NHS, feedback is not the sole implementation strategy, but those planning audits should avoid relying on feedback alone as the method for implementing change.

2 Feedback and other methods of implementation

The objective of this component of the overview was to determine the effectiveness of audit and feedback in comparison with other methods, and whether the addition of other methods improves impact. We identified 35 reviews of interventions that either included feedback used alone or in combination with other interventions, or compared feedback to other interventions (*see* Table 4.2 on CD-ROM).

Feedback

Feedback can be effective in improving prescribing by primary care physicians,[347] as part of training communication skills,[348] and feedback of costing information can change GP behaviour.[349] Feedback alone or in combination with other interventions can improve immunisation rates but the effect is variable.[350] Feedback can influence diagnostic and preventive performance in ambulatory care, but reminders appear to have more effect.[351] Thomson O'Brien *et al.* undertook a review to compare audit and feedback with other interventions and whether effectiveness could be improved by modifying how feedback is provided.[352] The limited evidence available did not indicate a measurable effect due to adding a complementary intervention to audit and feedback.

Educational interventions

The effects of continuing medical education (CME) are inconsistent,[353] and the evidence about impact in primary care settings is limited.[354] Educational interventions targeted at patients can improve the expression of treatment preferences at the end of life, and interventions targeted at physicians can increase the use of patient preferences, but sophisticated educational interventions may be required to change physician behaviour or the outcomes of care.[355] Educational outreach is a promising approach to implementing change in professional behaviour, especially prescribing.[356]

Opinion leaders

Thomson O'Brien *et al.* reviewed the effectiveness of opinion leaders. The eight studies identified indicated that the method does influence professional behaviour, but the changes were not always of practical importance.[357] The role and actions of the opinion leaders in different studies was not always clear, and the methods of delivering this intervention need clarifying.

Computer systems and reminders

Computerised information interventions (patient and physician reminders, treatment planners, and patient education) can improve aspects of care in family medicine.[358]

System changes

Organisational changes in primary care, such as nurse implementation of care protocols, multidisciplinary teams, or regional organisation of services improved aspects of care, but not health outcomes.[359] The effects of on site mental health workers in primary care are inconsistent but may have an effect on prescribing behaviour of primary care physicians when used with a multifaceted intervention.[360] The effects of the introduction of continuous quality improvement/total quality management are difficult to judge on the basis of current evidence.[361]

Incentives

Financial incentives can influence use of healthcare resources by professionals, but conclusions about the effect of combining feedback and incentives cannot be drawn because of the limited evidence available.[362]

Various methods compared

Traditional CME had little effect, feedback and opinion leaders have a moderate effect, but reminders, patient mediated interventions, academic detailing, and multifaceted interventions are more effective.[363–368] Methods to prompt physicians to follow the guidelines during the consultation are relatively powerful.[369] Reminders and feedback improved physician screening for cancer.[370] Computerised reminders and outreach can be effective in improving prescribing in primary care, and feedback may also be effective in certain types of prescribing.[371]

Printed educational materials such as guidelines alone have little effect, and the addition of feedback or workshops did not produce substantial changes, but outreach visits and opinion leaders were more likely to produce worthwhile improvements.[372] Printed educational materials were also less likely than reminders, feedback, or outreach to improve doctors' prescribing behaviour.[373] Lomas also reported that mailed educational materials are of little effect; combinations of interventions are generally more effective.[374] In a review of the implementation of guidelines in primary care using a variety of methods, little evidence was found to indicate that outcomes were improved,[375] and the impact of interventions may be influenced by the topic and setting.[353]

Education and the provision of information, learning through social influence, feedback, physician reminders, organisational interventions, and multifaceted interventions can be effective in improving the delivery of preventive services in primary care, but the effects are variable and generally small to moderate,[376] and more research is needed to determine factors that influence the effect of different interventions. Feedback, brief or intensive training, and multifaceted interventions had some effects in improving the diagnosis and treatment of mental disorders in primary care, but the available evidence is limited.[377] Multifaceted interventions can improve the performance of community professionals managing patients with diabetes, and organisational interventions that prompt regular recall and review also improve management.[378] Patient-oriented interventions such as patient education improved outcomes. In improving the use of diagnostic tests, education was of little effect, audit with feedback relatively weak, but administrative interventions can be effective.[379]

Discussion

The findings indicate that audit with feedback can be effective in changing performance, but as indicated in the reviews of feedback alone, the effects are variable and sometimes nil. In comparison with other interventions, it is more effective than traditional didactic education or mailings of educational material, but less effective than reminders, educational outreach, or multifaceted interventions. Changes to systems of care also appear to be potentially effective. However, the effects of all these interventions tend to vary with the topic or setting.

Thomson O'Brien *et al.* did not find that the addition of a complementary intervention to audit and feedback produced additional benefit.[352] However, the available evidence was limited. In contrast, multifaceted interventions, many of which included feedback, tended to be more effective. Several reviews, including the CRD overview, concluded that a multifaceted intervention designed to meet particular local circumstances was the most the appropriate approach to implementing change in performance in a clinical setting. Generalisable evidence of the effectiveness of this tailored approach to implementation may be difficult to obtain in randomised trials since local circumstances are highly variable.

Some of the limitations of the evidence should be noted. Although there is a growing number of trials of implementation methods, the studies do not adequately cover all types of health professionals and all clinical topics. For example, we did not identify reviews of studies of interventions to improve the technical performance of surgeons or the patient management skills of clinical psychologists. The reviews should be regarded as providing general guidance rather than concrete recommendations about the most effective interventions to employ.

3 Reviews of interventions other than audit and feedback

The objective of the third component of the overview was to identify effective interventions that could be used in the context of audit in the NHS. We identified 25 reviews of the effectiveness of interventions other than audit with feedback (*see* Table 4.3 on CD-ROM).

Reminders, computer support and decision aids

Reminders may be targeted at health professionals or patients. They may be delivered before or during a consultation, and by electronic, paper or other methods. Physician reminders can improve the proportion of patients receiving aspects of preventive healthcare.[382,383]

Computer-based reminder systems can improve the provision of preventive services in ambulatory care, although computer systems are not more effective than manual systems.[384] However, the combination of computer and manual reminders appeared to be superior to manual reminders alone. Computer-based guideline implementation systems may provide reminders, alerts, or recommendations. Guideline adherence can be improved by these systems, but improvement is variable and the impact on outcome is not clear.[385] When used in general practice, computer systems can improve performance, particularly preventive care.[386] However, consultation length increased and the benefits on outcome have not been adequately investigated.

Computer-based clinical decision support systems integrate patient-specific information and present results to clinicians. They can improve dosage decisions and reduce adverse drug reactions and length of stay among hospital patients receiving medication with a narrow therapeutic window, e.g. warfarin, nitroprusside, lignocaine.[387] Hunt *et al.* also reported that they can improve performance for drug dosing and preventive care, and may also improve other aspects of care including management of hypertension and diabetes, but evidence about the effects on outcome are limited.[388]

Colombet *et al.* undertook a review of decision aids for the triage of patients with chest pain, including computerised or non-computerised risk prediction models, decision rules or formalised triage protocols.[389] There were some benefits from the use of decision aids, including reduced length of hospital stay and improved sensitivity and specificity of diagnosis, but larger studies are required to determine any effect on mortality.

Education

Formal continuing medical education (CME) employs a variety of methods, including conferences, courses, meetings, symposia, lectures and clinical rounds. In a review of 14 studies, Davis *et al.* concluded that didactic sessions were not effective, although interactive sessions that provide the opportunity to practise skills can change professional performance, and occasionally outcomes.[390] Beaudry concluded that CME may improve physician knowledge and performance, and patient health status, but this review was not restricted to randomised trials.[391] However, generalisation may be hindered by inadequate evaluation methods and lack of comparability between programmes.[392] Continuing nursing education (CNE) does appear to have an effect on nursing practice, although the available evidence is limited.[393] A nursing record system is the record of care planned and/or given to patients by qualified nurses under the direction of a qualified nurse. The available evidence is insufficient to enable clear conclusions about the effectiveness of this method in influencing nursing performance.[394]

Training of health professionals in smoking cessation may be delivered in tutorials or workshops, or in personal tutorials.[395] The intensity of training and the methods used may vary. In a review of trials of smoking cessation training, professional performance improved, but smoking quit rates only increased in two of the eight included studies.

Outreach can be effective in improving the prescribing of some medications in nursing homes.[396]

There is insufficient evidence to determine the effectiveness of interprofessional education during which members of more than one health or social care profession learn together with the purpose of improving collaboration.[397] Furthermore, the effect of interventions to promote collaboration between nurses and doctors is unclear because the number of relevant studies is limited.[398]

Incentives

Evidence about the effects of target payments in primary care is insufficient to provide a clear answer as to whether this approach offers a method to improve performance.[399] There is some evidence that the method of payment affects the behaviour of primary care physicians, with fee-for-service systems resulting in more patient visits and greater continuity of care, but patients were less satisfied with access to their physician in comparison with salaried payments.[400] However, the generalisability of these findings is not clear.

Mass marketing
Media campaigns targeted at the population level are frequently used to promote or discourage the use of healthcare. Radio, television, newspapers, magazines, and leaflets may all be used. There is limited evidence, but that which is available indicates that mass media interventions do influence the use of healthcare interventions.[401]

Various methods compared
A small number of reviews considered several interventions, but not audit and feedback. In one, evidence was limited about the effects of interventions to improve health professionals' management of obese people.[402] There was also insufficient evidence about effect of different methods to improve outpatient referrals from general practice to hospital, including fundholding, joint consultant/general practitioner consulting sessions, local consensus meetings or educational seminars.[403] The dissemination and implementation of guidelines in professions allied to medicine does appear to have an effect, but evidence is limited and the comparative impact of different implementation methods cannot be determined.[174]

The subject of a practice guideline may influence the extent to which its recommendations are followed.[404,405] Adherence to high complexity recommendations was lower than for low complexity recommendations, complexity being determined from the degree of uncertainty about a procedure and the physician's control over the required resources. Recommendations that could be tested beforehand by physicians (high trialability) were also more likely to be adhered to.

Discussion
The findings of this component of the overview largely reinforce the findings of the overview of reviews of audit and feedback and other interventions. Mass marketing and incentives have been identified as additional potentially effective interventions, but these are not readily employed within the context of clinical audit. The potential of interactive education and outreach is reiterated, and reviews of reminder systems confirm they can be effective. Computer-based decision support and decision aids can also be effective in some circumstances.

Conclusions

We sought to determine (a) whether audit with feedback alone could lead to clinically useful improvements in the process and/or outcome of care; (b) the effectiveness of audit with feedback alone in comparison with other methods; (c) whether the addition of other methods improves the impact of feedback; and (d) whether other effective interventions could be used in the context of audit in the NHS.

A large body of evidence is now available from systematic reviews of methods of implementing change in performance, and general conclusions may be drawn. Audit with feedback can lead to clinically useful improvements in care, but the effect is variable. Sometimes the effect is nil. Some other methods can be more effective, including reminders and outreach visits. However, no single method can be relied on to be effective for all topics and in all circumstances. Multifaceted interventions tend to be more effective, and therefore in undertaking clinical audit, a variety of interventions should be selected in accordance with local circumstances and the topic. Feedback will be one element of the plan since it will be necessary to monitor the impact, but feedback alone cannot be relied upon to implement change.

Interactive education, outreach visits, reminder systems, decision aids, and system changes may all be considered as possible elements of a multifaceted intervention since there is evidence to show that they can be effective.

Key points

- Those planning audits should avoid relying on feedback alone as the method for implementing change; although feedback of data alone can occasionally be effective, change is much more likely if it forms part of a more complex set of change processes/interventions.
- The dissemination of educational materials, such as guidelines, has little effect unless accompanied by the use of selected implementation methods.
- Interactive educational interventions including outreach, service user and/or professional reminders (whether manual or computerised), decision support, and system change can sometimes, but not always, be effective.
- In audit, the use of multifaceted interventions chosen to suit the particular circumstances is more likely to be effective in changing performance than the use of a single intervention alone.

5 Discussion and conclusions

Limitations of the reviews

The limitations of the reviews should be considered first. It has already been made clear that we have not undertaken a systematic review and the findings should be viewed with this point in mind.

The reviews of methods of audit and the organisation of projects and programmes identified and included a large number of articles, but some articles may have been overlooked. Reports of many audits are not published in journals, and although we hand searched several journals, we will have failed to include audits published in other non-indexed journals, or in reports and other unofficial documents. Our search strategies concentrated on audit, and excluded other quality improvement methods. There are many publications relevant to quality improvement methods that will have been omitted, and it should be noted that the term audit is used in the UK to apply to a wider range of activities than in many other countries. Therefore, the articles included a large proportion from the UK. Furthermore, we did not seek articles published before 1996, since the NCCA review included articles up to 1996.

The review of the organisation of audit concentrated on audit in the UK. Articles reporting evaluation of quality improvement programmes in other countries were omitted since characteristics of different healthcare systems and the quality improvement systems in use would raise questions about the relevance of the findings to the UK system. Nevertheless, there might have been some general conclusions of relevance.

However, despite these qualifications a large number of articles were identified relating to methods and organisation of audit and consistent findings emerged. Therefore, the review can be regarded as providing useful guidance about the conduct of audit.

The review of systematic reviews built on the CRD review and is likely to have included most relevant reviews, and the original studies included in the review were generally randomised trials. However, since we did not review the original trials included in the reviews, the details of use of the implementation method in each study could not be studied.

General conclusions

The conclusions are summarised by the key points. These are duplicated in *Principles for Best Practice in Clinical Audit* and are intended to provide practical advice about audit.

A key finding is that the issues identified in relation to implementing change in audit, the organisation of audit projects and audit programmes, and the findings of the systematic reviews of studies of implementation methods indicate similar conclusions. The successful implementation of improvements in healthcare depends in large measure on a conducive environment within healthcare organisations that includes the promotion of positive attitudes and provision of the time and resources required. Leadership and effective teamwork are important organisational attributes. Audit teams in particular require support and training. There is adequate evidence about the methods of audit, including projects that should encourage greater involvement of users, the use of more systematic methods of selecting criteria and collecting data, and the use of a variety of approaches to suit the setting and topic concerned.

Effective implementation usually requires the use of a multifaceted intervention, chosen following an assessment of local circumstances. Thus staff undertaking audit should be willing to devote time and effort to creating implementation plans.

Issues for future research

The reviews also point to issues for future research, and since patients should be involved in audit, their involvement in setting priorities for research in this field is recommended. On the basis of this review, however, the following suggestions are made.

An important issue in need of further study is how healthcare organisations can be enabled to create an environment that facilitates audit and quality improvement. Many studies and reports of audits highlighted the relationship between the organisation and its staff as crucial to the success of efforts to change practice, but there were few reports of interventions designed to influence organisational behaviour. In particular, information about effective and practical methods of supporting audit teams, and healthcare teams in general, is required.

A review of the role of standard setting and benchmarking for UK healthcare organisations would be justified. There is limited information on this issue in the UK, but some countries have more experience.

Although the measurement of outcomes has been investigated extensively, the methods of adjusting for case mix are limited to a small number of settings. A review of case mix adjustment would be justified.

The new quality improvement techniques, in particular rapid-cycle data collection, are being introduced, and evidence is needed about the effectiveness of these methods, how they can be best applied, and the circumstances in which they are most effective.

6 References

1 NICE. *Principles for Best Practice in Clinical Audit*. Oxford, Radcliffe Medical Press, 2002.

2 Dixon, N. *Good Practice in Clinical Audit. A summary of selected literature to support criteria for clinical audit*. London, National Centre for Clinical Audit, 1996.

3 NHS Centre for Reviews and Dissemination. Getting evidence into practice. *Effective Health Care* 1999; **5**(1).

4 Bhatti-Sinclair K, Wheal A. Analysis of the external audit on ethnically sensitive practice. *Journal of Clinical Effectiveness* 1998; **3**: 6–9.

5 Bailey CC, Sparrow JM, Grey RH, Cheng H. The National Diabetic Retinopathy Laser Treatment Audit. I. Maculopathy. *Eye* 1998; **12**: 69–76.

6 Lunn JN. The history and achievements of the National Confidential Enquiry into Perioperative Deaths. *Journal of Quality in Clinical Research* 1998; **18**: 29–35.

7 Sharp JF, Forsyth DR. Audit of prescribing safety in a department of medicine for the elderly. *Journal of Clinical Effectiveness* 1996; **1**: 22–4.

8 Simmonds M, Edwards P. Pain relief in the recovery room: An audit of current practice and a proposed solution. *Journal of Clinical Effectiveness* 1998; **3**: 122–7.

9 Sharma SV, Fortes Mayer G. Cervical smears technique: re-audit. *Audit Trends* 1998; **6**: 23.
10 Dearlove J. Being kind to babies: An audit of paediatric radiology for first urinary infections. *British Journal of Clinical Governance* 1999; **4**: 7–10.
11 Kendall JM, McCabe SE. The use of audit to set up a thrombolysis programme in the accident and emergency department. *Emergency Medicine Journal* 1996; **13**: 49–53.
12 Srinivasan V, Sherman IW, O'Sullivan G. Surgical management of intractable epistaxis: Audit of results. *Journal of Laryngology & Otology* 2000; **114**: 697–700.
13 Dunn C. Clinically effective leg ulcer care. (Promoting Action for Clinical Effectiveness series). *Nursing Times* 1998; –3.
14 Turner P, Whitfield A, Brewster S, Halligan M, Kennedy J. The assessment of pain: An audit of physiotherapy practice. *Australian Journal of Physiotherapy* 1996; **42**: 55–62.
15 Gladstone J, Sutherland S. Focusing on risk: a simple audit study can have a major impact on clinical practice. *Journal of Clinical Effectiveness* 1997; **2**: 6–9.
16 Free C, Dawe A, Macey S, Mawer C. Evaluating and developing contraceptive services: The results of an audit of the North Lambeth Primary Care Commissioning Group. *British Journal of Family Planning* 2001; **27**: 22–8.
17 Khunti K, Goyder E, Baker R. Collation and comparison of multi-practice audit data: prevalence and treatment of known diabetes mellitus. *British Journal of General Practice* 1999; **49**: 375–9.
18 Dowson LJ, Mushtaq M, Watts T, Shurvinton J, Gooch R, Hayton R *et al.* A re-audit of pulmonary function laboratories in the West Midlands. *Respiratory Medicine* 1998; **92**: 1155–62.
19 Hayes S, Stewart K. The role of audit in making do not resuscitate decisions. *Journal of Evaluation in Clinical Practice* 1999; **5**: 305–12.
20 Holden JD. A short audit of folic acid prophylaxis for women with epilepsy. *Journal of Clinical Excellence* 1999; **1**: 75–7.
21 Holden J, Myles S, Skinner A. A district-wide audit and evaluation of palliative care services for 683 patients. *Journal of Clinical Governance* 2000; **8**: 31–6.
22 Joshi G, Landers DF. Audit in transfusion practice. *Journal of Evaluation* 1998; **4**: 141–6.
23 Nightingale J, Hargreaves J. An audit of incoming and outgoing medical records. *Audit Trends* 1996; **4**: 11–23.
24 Howe A. Can GPs audit their ability to detect psychological distress? One approach and some unresolved issues. *British Journal of General Practice* 1998; **48**: 899–902.
25 Hardern RD. Effective care of acute asthma in the Accident and Emergency department. *Journal of Evaluation in Clinical Practice* 1999; **5**: 93–6.
26 Mudge K, Braidwood L. Out of hours service reduces stress levels in general practitioners. *Journal of Clinical Governance* 1999; **7**: 48–51.
27 Smith AJ, Preston D. Communications between professional groups in an NHS trust hospital. *Journal of Management in Medicine* 1996; **10**: 31–9.

28 Institute of Medicine. Guidelines for clinical practice: From development to use. Washington DC: National Academic Press, 1992.
29 Baker R, Fraser RC. Development of review criteria: linking guidelines and assessment of quality. *British Medical Journal* 1995; **311**: 370–3.
30 AHCPR. Using clinical practice guidelines to evaluate quality of care. Rockville MD: US Department of Health & Human Services, 1995.
31 Bhatti-Sinclair K, Wheal A. Using external audit to review ethnically sensitive practice. *Journal of Clinical Effectiveness* 1998; **3**: 2–5.
32 Prvulovich EM, Jarritt PH, Vivian GC, Clarke SE, Pennell DJ, Underwood SR. Quality assurance in myocardial perfusion tomography: A collaborative BNCS/BNMS audit programme. *Nuclear Medicine Communications* 1998; **19**: 831–8.
33 Corben V. The Buckinghamshire nursing record audit tool: a unique approach to documentation. *Journal of Nursing Management* 1997; **5**: 289–93.
34 Naylor CD, Guyatt GH. Users' guides to the medical literature. XI. How to use an article about a clinical utilization review. Evidence-Based Medicine Working Group. *Journal of the American Medical Association* 1996; **275**: 1435–9.
35 Hofer TP, Hayward RA, Greenfield S, Wagner EH, Kaplan SH, Manning WG. The unreliability of individual physician "report cards" for assessing the costs and quality of care of a chronic disease. *Journal of the American Medical Association* 1999; **281**: 2098–105.
36 van Walraven C, Naylor CD. Do we know what inappropriate laboratory utilization is? A systematic review of laboratory clinical audits. *Journal of the American Medical Association* 1998; **280**: 550–8.
37 Ryan AA, Logue HF. Developing an audit tool for primary nursing. *Journal of Clinical Nursing* 1998; **7**: 417–23.
38 James PA, Cowan TM, Graham RP, Majeroni BA, Fox CH, Jaen CR. Using a clinical practice guideline to measure physician practice: translating a guideline for the management of heart failure. *Journal of the American Board of Family Practice* 1997; **10**: 206–12.
39 Johnson L, Hunt J, Burns C. Clinical effectiveness works: a practical approach to the assessment of leg ulcers. *Journal of Clinical Excellence* 1999; **1**: 59–63.
40 Sheikh A. Pneumococcal Vaccination: a Practice Based Audit. *Audit Trends* 1998; **6**: 93–5.
41 Fraser RC, Khunti K, Baker R, Lakhani M. Effective audit in general practice: a method for systematically developing audit protocols containing evidence-based review criteria. *British Journal of General Practice* 1997; **47**: 743–6.
42 Hadorn DC, Baker DW, Kamberg CJ, Brooks RH. Phase II of the AHCPR-sponsored heart failure guideline: translating practice recommendations into review criteria. *Joint Commission Journal on Quality Improvement* 1996; **22**: 265–76.
43 Cluzeau FA, Littlejohns P, Grimshaw JM, Feder G, Moran SE. Development and application of a generic methodology to assess the quality of clinical guidelines. *International Journal for Quality in Health Care* 1999; **11**: 21–8.

44 Rudkin A, Heason C, Rowe D. An audit of health monitoring in an adult population with profound learning disability. *Journal of Clinical Excellence* 1999; **1**: 137–40.
45 Poole P, Johnson S. Integrated care pathways: an orthopaedic experience. *Physiotherapy* 1996; **82**: 28–30.
46 Kitchiner D, Davidson C, Bundred P. Integrated Care Pathways: effective tools for continuous evaluation of clinical practice. *Journal of Evaluation in Clinical Practice* 1996; **2**: 65–9.
47 Birchall MA. Consensus standards for the process of cancer care: a modified expert panel method applied to head and neck cancer. South and West Expert Tumour Panel for Head and Neck Cancer. *British Journal of Cancer* 1998; **77**: 1926–31.
48 Layton A, Moss F, Morgan G. Mapping out the patient's journey: experiences of developing pathways of care. *Quality in Health Care* 1998; **7(suppl)**: s30–36.
49 Memel DS, Turton P, Rimmer JW. The care of disabled people in primary care. *Journal of Clinical Governance* 1999; **7**: 79–83.
50 Grimshaw GM, Baker R, Wilson AD, Thompson JR. Screening for diabetic retinopathy; towards a model for the evaluation and planning of screening programmes. *Journal of Clinical Excellence* 1999; **1**: 41–6.
51 Hutchinson A, McIntosh A, Anderson JP, Gilbert CL and Field R. *Evidence based review criteria for Type 2 diabetes foot care*. Sheffield, RCGP Effective Clinical Practice Unit, University of Sheffield, 2000.
52 Campbell SM, Roland MO, Shekelle PG, Cantrill SA, Buetow SA, Cragg DK. Development of review criteria for assessing the quality of management of non-insulin dependent diabetes mellitus in general practice. *Quality in Health Care* 1999; **8**: 6–15.
53 Harrison M, Johnston S, Heathcote J. Agreeing consensus and maintaining enthusiasm for district-wide audit: Bromley MAAG's experience of auditing diabetes care. *Journal of Clinical Governance* 1999; **7**: 74–8.
54 Normand SL, McNeil BJ, Peterson LE, Palmer RH. Eliciting expert opinion using the Delphi technique: identifying performance indicators for cardiovascular disease. *International Journal for Quality in Health Care* 1998; **10**: 247–60.
55 Vanderpump MP, Ahlquist JA, Franklyn JA, Clayton RN. Consensus statement for good practice and audit measures in the management of hypothyroidism and hyperthyroidism. The Research Unit of the Royal College of Physicians of London, the Endocrinology and Diabetes Committee of the Royal College of Physicians of London, and the Society for Endocrinology. *British Medical Journal* 1996; **313**: 539–44.
56 Bateman DN. Clearing 'the fog on the Tyne': can the quality of therapeutics be assessed? *Clinical & Experimental Pharmacology & Physiology* 1996; **23**: 1005–9.
57 Jamieson M, Griffiths R, Jayasuriya R. Developing outcomes for community nursing: the Nominal Group Technique. *Australian Journal of Advanced Nursing* 1998; **16**: 14–9.

58 Murphy MK, Black NA, Lamping DL, McKee CM, Sanderson CF, Askham J *et al*. Consensus development methods, and their use in clinical guideline development. *Health Technology Assessment (South Hampton, NY)* 1998; **2**: i–iv.

59 Shekelle PG, Kahan JP, Bernstein SJ, Leape LL, Kamberg CJ, Park RE. The reproducibility of a method to identify the overuse and underuse of medical procedures. *New England Journal of Medicine* 1998; **338**: 1888–95.

60 Berlowitz DR, Ash AS, Hickey EC, Friedman RH, Kader B, Moskowitz MA. Outcomes of hypertension care. Simple measures are not that simple. *Medical Care* 1997; **35**: 742–6.

61 Goodacre SW, Gillett M, Harris RD, Houlihan KP. Consistency of retrospective triage decisions as a standardised instrument for audit. *Emergency Medicine Journal* 1999; **16**: 322–4.

62 Lubrano E, Butterworth M, Hesselden A, Wells S, Helliwell P. An audit of anthropometric measurements by medical and physiotherapy staff in patients with ankylosing spondylitis. *Clinical Rehabilitation* 1998; **12**: 216–20.

63 Baker R, Fraser RC. Is ownership more important than the scientific credibility of audit protocols? A survey of medical audit advisory groups. *Family Practice* 1997; **14**: 107–11.

64 Elwyn G, Currie J, Rapport FL, Kirby A, Koppel SM. A shared confusion? An audit of lithium monitoring in an inner city general practice. A short report. *Audit Trends* 1997; **5**: 85–9.

65 Libeer JC. Total quality management for clinical laboratories: a need or a new fashion? *Acta Clinica Belgica* 1997; **52**: 226–32.

66 Martimo KP. Audit matrix for evaluating Finnish occupational health units. *Scandinavian Journal of Work, Environment & Health* 1998; **24**: 439–43.

67 Cryer HG, Hiatt JR, Fleming AW, Gruen JP, Sterling J. Continuous use of standard process audit filters has limited value in an established trauma system. *Journal of Trauma-Injury Infection & Critical Care* 1996; **41**: 389–94.

68 Kiefe CI, Weissman NW, Allison JJ, Farmer R, Weaver M, Williams OD. Identifying achievable benchmarks of care: concepts and methodology. *International Journal for Quality in Health Care* 1998; **10**: 443–7.

69 Allison J, Kiefe CI, Weissman NW. Can data-driven benchmarks be used to set the goals of healthy people 2010? *American Journal of Public Health* 1999; **89**: 61–5.

70 Weissman NW, Allison JJ, Kiefe CI, Farmer RM, Weaver MT, Williams OD *et al*. Achievable benchmarks of care: the ABCs of benchmarking. *Journal of Evaluation in Clinical Practice* 1999; **5**: 269–81.

71 Clark JD, Kerr WJ, Davis MH. CASES – clinical audit; scenarios for evaluation and study. *British Dental Journal* 1997; **183**: 108–11.

72 Drachman DA. Benchmarking patient satisfaction at academic health centers. *Joint Commission Journal on Quality Improvement* 1996; **22**: 359–67.

73 Fitzgerald RP, Shiverick BN, Zimmerman D. Applying performance measures to long-term care. *Joint Commission Journal on Quality Improvement* 1996; **22**: 505–17.

74 Martin R, Fodor J. Benchmarking in radiation oncology: discovering inconsistencies in reporting methodologies. *Administrative Radiology Journal* 1997; **16**: 31–4.
75 Thomson RG, McElroy H, Kazandjian VA. Maryland Hospital Quality Indicator Project in the United Kingdom: an approach for promoting continuous quality improvement. *Quality in Health Care* 1997; **6**: 49–55.
76 Wells CA, Perera R, White FE, Domizio P. Fine needle aspiration cytology in the UK breast screening programme: A national audit of results. *Breast* 1999; **8**: 261–6.
77 Penney GC, Pearson D. A national audit to monitor the uptake of clinical guidelines on the management of diabetes in pregnancy. *Journal of Clinical Governance* 2000; **5**: 28–34.
78 Maceneaney PM, Malone DE, Skehan SJ, Curry MP, Miller JC, Gibney RG *et al*. The role of hepatic arterial doppler ultrasound after liver transplantation: An 'Audit Cycle' evaluation. *Clinical Radiology* 2000; **55**: 517–24.
79 Schreuder F, Powell BWE. Incomplete excision of basal cell carcinomas: An audit. *British Journal of Clinical Governance* 1999; **4**: 43–4.
80 Butler C, Smithers M, Stott N, Peters J. Audit-enhanced, district-wide primary care for people with diabetes mellitus. *European Journal of General Practice* 1997; **3**: 23–7.
81 Hutchings D. Evaluating multidisciplinary teams: an example of an audit framework. *British Journal of Therapy & Rehabilitation* 1996; **3**: 371–2, 389–90.
82 Scott F, Newens A. Hospital monitoring of pressure ulcers in the UK. *Journal of Wound Care* 1999; **8**: 221–4.
83 Crombie IK, Davies HTO. Beyond health outcomes: the advantages of measuring process. *Journal of Evaluation in Clinical Practice* 1998; **4**: 31–8.
84 Marek KD. Measuring the effectiveness of nursing care. *Outcomes Management for Nursing Practice* 1997; **1**: 8–12.
85 Brook RH, McGlynn EA, Cleary PD. Quality of healthcare. Part 2: measuring quality of care. *New England Journal of Medicine* 1996; **335**: 966–70.
86 Palmer RH. Using health outcomes data to compare plans, networks and providers. *International Journal for Quality in Health Care* 1998; **10**: 477–83.
87 Mant J, Hicks NR. Assessing quality of care: what are the implications of the potential lack of sensitivity of outcome measures to differences in quality? *Journal of Evaluation in Clinical Practice* 1996; **2**: 243–8.
88 Freeman JA, Playford ED, Nicholas RS, Thompson AJ. A neurological rehabilitation unit: audit of activity and outcome. *Journal of the Royal College of Physicians of London* 1996; **30**: 21–6.
89 Mark H, Garet DE. Interpreting profiling data in behavioral healthcare for a continuous quality improvement cycle. *Joint Commission Journal on Quality Improvement* 1997; **23**: 521–8.
90 McColl A, Roderick P, Gabbay J, Ferris G. What do health authorities think of population based health outcome indicators? *Quality in Health Care* 1998; **7**: 90–7.
91 McGivney WT, Barker ML, Bost JE, Burns J, Loeb JM, Morris M *et al*. Panel discussion. Data needs in cancer. *Oncology* 1998; **12**: 147–56.

92 McMillan TM, Sparkes C. Goal planning and neurorehabilitation: The Wolfson Neurorehabilitation Centre Approach. *Neuropsychological Rehabilitation* 1999; **9**: 241–51.

93 Rainwater JA, Romano PS, Antonius DM. The California Hospital Outcomes Project: how useful is California's report card for quality improvement? *Joint Commission Journal on Quality Improvement* 1998; **24**: 31–9.

94 Rocke DA, Arsiradam NM. The difficult airway in obstetrics. *Current Opinion in Anaesthesiology* 1997; **10**: 176–80.

95 Sakallaris BR, Jastremski CA, Von Rueden KT. Clinical decision support systems for outcome measurement and management. *AACN Clinical Issues* 2000; **11**: 351–62.

96 Semmens JB, Lawrence-Brown M, Fletcher DR, Rouse IL, Holman CDJ. The quality of surgical care project: A model to evaluate surgical outcomes in western Australia using population-based record linkage. *Australian & New Zealand Journal of Surgery* 1998; **68**: 397–403.

97 O'Donnell A, Tucker L. Pre-dialysis education. A change in clinical practice. How effective is it? *Edtna-Erca Journal* 1999; **25**: 29–32.

98 Khuri SF, Daley J, Henderson W, Hur K, Demakis J, Aust JB *et al.* The Department of Veterans Affairs' NSQIP: the first national, validated, outcome-based, risk-adjusted, and peer-controlled program for the measurement and enhancement of the quality of surgical care. National VA Surgical Quality Improvement Program. *Annals of Surgery* 1998; **228**: 491–507.

99 Prytherch DR, Whiteley MS, Higgins B, Weaver PC, Prout WG, Powell SJ. POSSUM and Portsmouth POSSUM for predicting mortality. *British Journal of Surgery* 1998; **85**: 1217–20.

100 Bardsley M, Cleary R. Assessing the outcomes of total knee replacement. *Journal of Evaluation in Clinical Practice* 1999; **5**: 47–55.

101 Brooker C, Molyneux P, Deverill M, Repper J. Evaluating clinical outcome and staff morale in a rehabilitation team for people with serious mental health problems. *Journal of Advanced Nursing* 1999; **29**: 44–51.

102 Long F, Dixon P. Monitoring outcomes in routine practice: defining appropriate measurement criteria. *Journal of Evaluation in Clinical Practice* 1996; **2**: 71–8.

103 Corbanese U, Possamai C, Casagrande L, Bordino P. Evaluation of trauma care: validation of the TRISS method in an Italian ICU. *Intensive Care Medicine* 1996; **22**: 941–6.

104 Fallon WF, Jr., Barnoski AL, Mancuso CL, Tinnell CA, Malangoni MA. Benchmarking the quality-monitoring process: a comparison of outcomes analysis by trauma and injury severity score (TRISS) methodology with the peer-review process. *Journal of Trauma-Injury Infection & Critical Care* 1997; **42**: 810–5.

105 Kingston R, O'Flanagan SJ. Scoring systems in trauma. *Irish Journal of Medical Science* 2000; **169**: 168–72.

106 Mead D, Moseley MA. Research based measurement tools in the audit process: issues of use, validity, and reliability. *Nurse Researcher* 1996; **3**: 185–202.

107 Richardson D, Tarnow-Mordi WO, Lee SK. Risk adjustment for quality improvement. *Pediatrics* 1999; **103**: 255–65.

108 Bakken S, Dolter KJ, Holzemer WL. A comparison of three strategies for risk-adjustment of outcomes for AIDS patients hospitalized for Pneumocystis carinii pneumonia. *Journal of Advanced Nursing* 1999; **30**: 1424–31.

109 Berlowitz DR, Ash AS, Hickey EC, Kader B, Friedman R, Moskowitz MA. Profiling outcomes of ambulatory care: casemix affects perceived performance. *Medical Care* 1998; **36**: 928–33.

110 Siegel C, Davis-Chambers E, Haugland G, Bank R, Aponte C, McCombs H. Performance measures of cultural competency in mental health organizations. *Administration & Policy in Mental Health* 2000; **28**: 91–106.

111 Papiernik E, Bucourt M, Zeitlin J. Measuring the success of the audit process: Results from the Seine-Saint-Denis perinatal audit. *Prenatal & Neonatal Medicine* 2000; **5**: 303–10.

112 Dixon J, Sanderson C, Elliott P, Walls P, Jones J, Petticrew M. Assessment of the reproducibility of clinical coding in routinely collected hospital activity data: a study in two hospitals. *Journal of Public Health Medicine* 1998; **20**: 63–9.

113 Hutchison T, Harpin V. Survey of UK computerised special needs registers. *Archives of Disease in Childhood* 1998; **78**: 312–5.

114 Paltiel O, Ronen I, Polliack A, Iscovich J, Epstein L. The contribution of multiple data sources to a clinical audit of lymphoma in a teaching hospital. *International Journal for Quality in Health Care* 1998; **10**: 303–9.

115 Del Mar C, Lowe JB, Adkins P, Arnold E. What is the quality of general practitioner records in Australia? *Australian Family Physician* 1996; **Suppl 1**: S21–S25.

116 Hale CA, Thomas LH, Bond S, Todd C. The nursing record as a research tool to identify nursing interventions. *Journal of Clinical Nursing* 1997; **6**: **207–14.**

117 Luck J, Peabody JW, Dresselhaus TR, Lee M, Glassman P. How well does chart abstraction measure quality? A prospective comparison of standardized patients with the medical record. *American Journal of Medicine* 2000; **108**: 642–9.

118 Sulmasy DP, Dwyer M, Marx E. Do the ward notes reflect the quality of end-of-life care? *Journal of Medical Ethics* 1996; **22**: 344–8.

119 Harwood P, Yeomans D. Inconsistencies in risk assessment. *Psychiatric Bulletin* 1998; **22**: 446–9.

120 Hermida J, Nicholas DD, Blumenfeld SN. Comparative validity of three methods for assessment of the quality of primary healthcare. *International Journal for Quality in Health Care* 1999; **11**: 429–33.

121 Vrancken Peeters MP, Kappetein AP, Lardenoye JH, Breslau PJ. The value of a mortality-scoring system in the quality control of patients undergoing abdominal aortic surgery. *European Journal of Vascular & Endovascular Surgery* 1999; **18**: 523–6.

122 Chasteen JE, Cameron CA, Phillips SL. An audit system for assessing dental record keeping. *Journal of Dental Education* 1996; **60**: 978–86.

123 Munck AP, Gahm-Hansen B, Sogaard P, Sogaard J. Long-lasting improvement in general practitioners' prescribing of antibiotics by means of medical audit. *Scandinavian Journal of Primary Health Care* 1999; **17**: 185–90.
124 Addison J, Tripathi P, Williams O, Richards HK, Pickard JD, Kirkpatrick PJ. Regional survey of the management of patients with transient ischaemic attacks. *Audit Trends* 1997; **5**: 35–8.
125 Lambert AW, O'Kelly F, Ranaboldo CJ. Analgesia for appendicitis. *Audit Trends* 1999; **7**: 19–21.
126 Rethans J-J, Westin S, Hays R. Methods for quality assessment in general practice. *Family Practice* 1996; **13**: 468–76.
127 Weingart SN, Iezzoni LI, Davis RB, Palmer RH, Cahalane M, Hamel MB *et al.* Use of administrative data to find substandard care: validation of the complications screening program. *Medical Care* 2000; **38**: 796–806.
128 Bader JD, Shugars DA, White BA, Rindal DB. Evaluation of audit-based performance measures for dental care plans. *Journal of Public Health Dentistry* 1999; **59**: 150–7.
129 Bader JD, Shugars DA, White BA, Rindal DB. Development of effectiveness of care and use of services measures for dental care plans. *Journal of Public Health Dentistry* 1999; **59**: 142–9.
130 Geraci JM, Ashton CM, Kuykendall DH, Johnson ML, Wu L. International Classification of Diseases, 9th Revision, Clinical Modification codes in discharge abstracts are poor measures of complication occurrence in medical inpatients. *Medical Care* 1997; **35**: 589–602.
131 Dresser MV, Feingold L, Rosenkranz SL, Coltin KL. Clinical quality measurement. Comparing chart review and automated methodologies. *Medical Care* 1997; **35**: 539–52.
132 Adhiyaman V, Oke A, White AD, Shah IU. Diagnoses in discharge communications: how far are they reliable? *International Journal of Clinical Practice* 2000; **54**: 457–8.
133 Gleeson CM, Reynolds F. Accidental dural puncture rates in UK obstetric practice. *International Journal of Obstetric Anesthesia* 1998; **7**: 242–6.
134 Walshe K. Adverse events in healthcare: issues in measurement. *Quality in Health Care* 2000; **9**: 47–52.
135 Bowers L. Monitoring the outcome of case management and community care: the care programme approach support system (CPASS). *Journal of Psychiatric & Mental Health Nursing* 1997; **4**: 37–44.
136 Munck AP, Gilsa HD, Lindman A, Ovhed I, Forre S, Torsteinsson JB. A Noridc collaboration on medical audit. The APO method for quality development and continuous medical education (CME) in primary healthcare. *Scandinavian Journal of Primary Health Care* 1998; **16**: 2–6.
137 Phillips W. Data collection in continence care. (Promoting Action on Clinical Effectiveness series. Evaluating outcomes of continence care). *Nursing Times* 1998; –60.

138 Wade JP, Weyman JC, Goldstone KE. CT standard protocols are of limited value in assessing actual patient dose. *British Journal of Radiology* 1997; **70**: 1146–51.

139 Thornton CM, O'Hara MD. A regional audit of perinatal and infant autopsies in Northern Ireland. *British Journal of Obstetrics & Gynaecology* 1998; **105**: 18–23.

140 Killick S. An audit spiral of subfertility referrals from primary care: strategies for improving quality of information. *Journal of Clinical Governance* 1999; **7**: 57–61.

141 Anderson GM, Beers MH, Kerluke K. Auditing prescription practice using explicit criteria and computerized drug benefit claims data. *Journal of Evaluation in Clinical Practice* 1997; **3**: 283–94.

142 Hughes LM, Holden JD, Tree AM. Audit as a method of reducing benzodiazepine prescribing in general practice. *Journal of Clinical Effectiveness* 1997; **2**: 79–82.

143 Brooker D. The efficacy of Dementia Care Mapping as an audit tool: Report of a 3-year British NHS evaluation. *Aging & Mental Health* 1999; **2**.

144 Tourish D, Mulholland J. Communication between nurses and nurse managers: a case study from an NHS Trust. *Journal of Nursing Management* 1997; **5**: 25–36.

145 Mead DM, Moseley LG, Cook RM. Can feedback be individualised, useful, and economical? *International Journal of Nursing Studies* 1997; **34**: 285–94.

146 Banks NJ. Designing medical record abstraction forms. *International Journal for Quality in Health Care* 1998; **10**: 163–7.

147 Bjorvell C, Thorell-Ekstrand I, Wredling R. Development of an audit instrument for nursing care plans in the patient record. *Quality in Health Care* 2000; **9**: 6–13.

148 Hopkins A, Irwin P, Wallace H. Conceptual differences amongst the data collection instruments used in clinical audit. *Journal of Evaluation in Clinical Practice* 1996; **2**: 153–8.

149 Beake S, McCourt C, Page L, Vail A. The use of clinical audit in evaluating maternity services reform: a critical reflection. *Journal of Evaluation in Clinical Practice* 1998; **4**: 75–83.

150 Brocklehurst J, Dickinson E, Windsor J. Sequential audits of geriatric care: measuring change in structure and process and the contribution of clinical audit. *Journal of the Royal College of Physicians of London* 1998; **32**: 564–7.

151 Lorenzoni L, Da Cas R, Aparo UL. The quality of abstracting medical information from the medical record: the impact of training programmes. *International Journal for Quality in Health Care* 1999; **11**: 209–13.

152 Bradley G. An audit of anticoagulant guidelines: the relative influence of education, presentation and complexity of guidelines on compliance. *Journal of Clinical Effectiveness* 1998; **3**: 84–9.

153 Hocking GR, Niteckis VN, Cairns BJ, Hayman JA. Departmental audit in surgical anatomical pathology. *Pathology* 1997; **29**: 418–21.

154 McDermott FT, Cordner SM, Tremayne AB. Consultative Committee on Road Traffic Fatalities: Trauma audit methodology. *Australian & New Zealand Journal of Surgery* 2000; **70**: 710–21.
155 Bayliss V, Cherry M, Locke R, Salter L. Pathways for continence care: background and audit. *British Journal of Nursing* 2000; **9**: 590–6.
156 Benneyan JC. Use and interpretation of statistical quality control charts. *International Journal for Quality in Health Care* 1998; **10**: 69–73.
157 Jarvis P. Audit: Samples and sampling. *Audit Trends* 1996; **4**: 145–7.
158 Lagoe RJ. Basic statistics for clinical pathway evaluation. *Nursing Economics* 1998; **16**: 125–31.
159 Khunti K, Baker R, Adams S. How effective was your audit? A new method of reporting audit results of improvement in standards of care. *Journal of Clinical Excellence* 1999; **1**: 147–50.
160 *Data Protection Act 1998*. London, The Stationery Office Limited, 1998.
161 Strobl J, Cave E, Walley T. Data protection legislation: interpretation and barriers to research. *British Medical Journal* 2000; **321**: 890–2.
162 Abi AG. Measuring change in the NHS. (Promoting Action on Clinical Effectiveness series. Developing a framework for monitoring and evaluating the implementation and outcomes of clinical effectiveness initiatives.) *Nursing Times* 1998; –9.
163 Bowie P, Dougall A, Brown R, Marshall D. Turnaround time of in-patient discharge letters: a simple system of audit. *Health Bulletin* 1996; **54**: 438–40.
164 Dudgeon DJ, Harlos M, Clinch JJ. The Edmonton Symptom Assessment Scale (ESAS) as an audit tool. *Journal of Palliative Care* 1999; **15**: 14–9.
165 Griffiths J, Hutchings W. The wider implications of an audit of care plan documentation. *Journal of Clinical Nursing* 1999; **8**: 57–65.
166 Guly HR. A scale for measuring the severity of diagnostic errors in accident and emergency departments. *Emergency Medicine Journal* 1997; **14**: 290–2.
167 Smith AJ. Chart reviews made simple. *Nursing Management* 1996; **27**: 33–4.
168 Twaddle S, Liao XH, Turnbull D, Kohli H. Can information on breast pathology reports be used to audit the UK Breast Screening Programme? *Health Bulletin* 1996; **54**: 123–5.
169 Sharma SV, Fortes Mayer G. Audit of influenza vaccination to maximise health benefit and practice income. *Audit Trends* 1998; **6**: 132–6.
170 Smellie WS, Galloway MJ, Chinn D. Benchmarking general practice use of pathology services: a model for monitoring change. *Journal of Clinical Pathology* 2000; **53**: 476–80.
171 Cabana MD, Rand CS, Powe NR, Wu AW, Wilson MH, Abbound PA, Rubin HR. Why don't physicians follow clinical practice guidelines? *Journal of the American Medical Association* 1999; **282**(15): 1458–65.
172 Abi AG, Raine R. Planning for action. (PACE series. Promoting Action on Clinical Effectiveness programme. Overcoming barriers to changing professional practice.) *Nursing Times* 1998.

173 Ruston A, Lawes M. Implementing clinical effectiveness: generalising the findings of a project based approach to implementing clinical guidelines for the management of leg ulcers. *Audit Trends* 1999; **7**: 5–10.
174 Smith GJ, Dobson P, Lumley H. Implementation of evidence-based guidelines for *Helicobacter pylori* eradication in Gateshead general practice. *Journal of Clinical Excellence* 1999; **1**: 69–74.
175 Livesey JP, Berry P, Cossham T, Hodgson D, Monk JP. An audit of lost X-ray films on orthopaedic and trauma wards. *Journal of Clinical Effectiveness* 1996; **1**: 57–8.
176 Eagle M, Knott P. Venous leg ulceration; guidelines and audit. A health authority initiative. *Journal of Clinical Excellence* 1999; **1**: 65–8.
177 Humphris P, Littlejohns P. Implementing clinical guidelines: linking learning and clinical audit. *Audit Trends* 2000; **4**: 59–62.
178 Menon KV, Bates T. Out-of-hours – operating failure to close the audit cycle. *Journal of Clinical Effectiveness* 1997; **2**: 83–5.
179 Bonetti PO, Waeckerlin A, Schuepfer G, Frutiger A. Improving time-sensitive processes in the intensive care unit: the example of 'door-to-needle time' in acute myocardial infarction. *International Journal for Quality in Health Care* 2000; **12**: 311–7.
180 Beaumont B. Methadone prescribing in general practice. *Audit Trends* 1997; **5**: 90–2.
181 Baker J. Evidence-based practice in pressure sore reduction. *Nursing Times* 1998; **94**: 47–9.
182 Murray R, Pollock L, Turner G. National Depot Neuroleptic Audit Project: identification and implementation of good nursing practice. *Journal of Psychiatric & Mental Health Nursing* 1998; **5**: 221–2.
183 Cass H, Kugler B. Service evaluation and development: experience of a paediatric disability team. *Child: Care, Health & Development* 1999; **25**: 115–27.
184 Sheldon T. Promoting healthcare quality: What role performance indicators? *Quality in Health Care* 1998; **7**: S45–S50.
185 Colville RJI, Laing JHE, Murison MSC. Coding plastic surgery operations: An audit of performance using OPCS-4. *British Journal of Plastic Surgery* 2000; **53**: 420–2.
186 London MR, Klug CD. A framework for improving quality: using project study teams, Providence Health System tackles problem areas. *Health Progress* 1998; **79**: 56–60.
187 Stead J, Round A. Feedback of X-ray frequency: a controlled trial between primary care groups. *Journal of Clinical Excellence* 1999; **1**: 133–6.
188 Eaton KA, Fleming WG, Rich JL. A report of an evaluation of the pilot peer review scheme for general dental practitioners working in the general dental services in England. *British Dental Journal* 1998; **184**: 178–82.
189 Hastings A, Shepherd D. Improving diabetic eye care in the community: the use of an eye care co-operation card. *Audit Trends* 1998; **6**: 141–6.

190 Dunning M. Securing change: lessons from the PACE programme. (PACE series. Promoting Action in Clinical Effectiveness.) *Nursing Times* 1998; –2.

191 Dunning M, Abi AG, Gilbert D. Turning evidence into everyday practice. (Promoting Action for Clinical Effectiveness series.) *Nursing Times* 1998.

192 Geboers H, van der Horst M, Mokkink H, van Montfort P, van den Bosch W, van den Hoogen H *et al.* Setting up improvement projects in small scale primary care practices: feasilibity of a model for continuous quality improvement. *Quality in Health Care* 1999; **8**: 36–42.

193 Bradshaw C, Murray E. Improving the care of patients without spleens in a district. *Journal of Clinical Effectiveness* 1997; **2**: 47–9.

194 Cox S, Wilcock P, Young J. Improving the repeat prescribing process in a busy general practice. A study using continuous qualty improvement methodology. *Quality in Health Care* 1999; **8**: 119–25.

195 Hodgkin P, Eve R, Golton I, Munro J, Musson G. Changing clinical behaviour on a city-wide scale: lessons from the FACTS project. *Journal of Clinical Effectiveness* 1996; **1**: 8–10.

196 Giles PD, Cunnington AR, Payne M, Crothers DC, Walsh MS. Cholesterol reduction for the secondary prevention of coronary heart disease: A successful multi-disciplinary approach to implementing evidence-based treatment in a district general hospital. *Journal of Clinical Effectiveness* 1998; **3**: 156–60.

197 Overdyk FJ, Harvey SC, Fishman RL, Shippey F. Successful strategies for improving operating room efficiency at academic institutions. *Anesthesia & Analgesia* 1998; **86**: 896–906.

198 Gandhi TK, Puopolo AL, Dasse P, Haas JS, Bustin HR, Cook EF *et al.* Obstacles to collaborative quality improvement: the case of ambulatory general medical care. *International Journal for Quality in Health Care* 2000; **12**: 115–23.

199 Ferlie E, Wood M, Fitzgerald L. Some limits to evidence based medicine: a case study from elective orthopaedics. *Quality in Health Care* 1999; **8**: 99–107.

200 Robinson MB, Thompson E, Black NA. Evaluation of the effectiveness of guidelines, audit and feedback: improving the use of intravenous thrombolysis in patients with suspected acute myocardial infarction. *International Journal for Quality in Health Care* 1996; **8**: 211–22.

201 Davies C, Fletcher J, Szczepura A, Wilmot J. Factors influencing audit in general practice. *International Journal of Health Care Quality* 1996; **9**: 5–9.

202 Howitt A, Armstrong D. Implementing evidence based medicine in general practice: audit and qualitative study of antithrombotic treatment for atrial fibrillation. *British Medical Journal* 1999; **318**: 1324–7.

203 Glauber J, Goldmann DA, Homer CJ, Berwick DM. Reducing medical error through systems improvement: the management of febrile infants. *Pediatrics* 2000; **105**: 1330–2.

204 McNaughton M, Cavanagh S. Changing urine testing protocols through audit. *Nursing Times* 1998; **94**: 42–3.

205 Schaubhut RM, Jones C. A systems approach to medication error reduction. *Journal of Nursing Care Quality* 2000; **14**: 13–27.

206 Alemi F, Moore S, Headrick L, Neuhauser D, Hekelman F, Kizys N. Rapid improvement teams. *Joint Commission Journal on Quality Improvement* 1998; **24**: 119–29.

207 Lawrence M, Packwood T. Adapting total quality management for general practice: evaluation of a programme. *Quality in Health Care* 1996; **5**: 151–8.

208 Fraser R, Farooqi A, Sorrie R. Assessing the long term impact of a completed audit in general practice: a follow-up after 11 years. *Audit Trends* 1996; **4**: 125–8.

209 McCarthy MJ, Byrne G, Silverman SH. The setting up and implementation of a venous thromboembolism prophylaxis policy in clinical hospital practice. *Journal of Evaluation in Clinical Practice* 1998; **4**: 113–7.

210 Wolff AM. Limited adverse occurrence screening: using medical record review to reduce hospital adverse patient events. *Medical Journal of Australia* 1996; **164**: 458–61.

211 Ashford J, Eccles M, Bond S, Hall LA, Bond J. Improving healthcare through professional behaviour change: introducing a framework for identifying behavior change strategies. *British Journal of Clinical Governance* 1999; **4**(1): 14–23.

212 Grol R. Personal paper: Beliefs and evidence in changing clinical practice. *British Medical Journal* 1997; **315**: 418–21.

213 Moulding NT, Silagy CA, Weller DP. A framework for effective management of change in clinical practice: Dissemination and implementation of clinical practice guidelines. *Quality in Health Care* 1999; **8**: 177–83.

214 Sculpher M. Evaluating the cost-effectiveness of interventions designed to increase the utilization of evidence-based guidelines. *Family Practice* 2000; **17 Suppl 1**: S26–S31.

215 Dawson S, Sutherland K, Dopson S, Miller R. Changing clinical practice: views about the management of adult asthma. *Quality in Health Care* 1999; **8**: 253–61.

216 Garala M, Craig J, Lee J. Reducing general practitioner referral for lumbar spine X-ray. *Journal of Clinical Governance* 1999; **7**: 186–9.

217 Oswald N, Bateman H. Treating individuals according to evidence: why do primary care practitioners do what they do? *Journal of Evaluation in Clinical Practice* 2000; **6**: 139–48.

218 Robertson N, Baker R, Hearnshaw H. Changing the clinical behaviour of doctors – a psychological framework. *Quality in Health Care* 1996; **5**: 51–4.

219 Veldhuis M, Wigersma L, Okkes I. Deliberate departures from good general practice: a study of motives among Dutch general practitioners. *British Journal of General Practice* 1998; **48**: 1833–6.

220 Department of Health. *The New NHS: modern, dependable*. London, The Stationery Office, 1997.

221 Department of Health. *A First Class Service: Quality in the New NHS*. London, Department of Health, 1998.

222 NHS Executive. *The NHS Plan*. London, Department of Health, 2000.

223 Kelson M. *User Involvement: A guide to developing effective user involvement strategies in the NHS*. London, College of Health, 1997.
224 Kelson M. *National Sentinel Audits Involving Older People: A guide to involving older people in local audit activity*. London, College of Health, 1999.
225 Kelson M. *Promoting Patient Involvement in Clinical Audit: Practical guidance on achieving effective involvement*. London, College of Health, 1998.
226 Rajasekar D, Bigrigg A. Patient involvement in topic selection for audit. *Journal of Clinical Governance* 1999; **7**: 136–7.
227 Kelson M. User involvement in clinical audit: a review of developments and issues of good practice. *Journal of Evaluation in Clinical Practice* 1996; **2**: 97–109.
228 Kelson M, Redpath L. Promoting user involvement in clinical audit; surveys of audit committees in primary and secondary care. *Journal of Clinical Effectiveness* 1996; **1**: 14–8.
229 Parr JH, Bradshaw C, Broderick W, Courtenay H, Eccles M, Murray E *et al.* Improving the use of aspirin in myocardial infarction: A district strategy. *British Journal of Clinical Governance* 1999; **4**: 24–7.
230 Abba K, Webster J. Facilitating the Audit of Asthma Management – The Liverpool PCAG experience. *Audit Trends* 1998; **6**: 54–8.
231 Dunleavy P, Farmer P. Service quality audit: involving users and carers in the community. *Community Care Management & Planning* 1996; **4**(5): 175–8.
232 Sehdev SS, Wilson A. Hospital care given in the event of a miscarriage: Views of women and their partners, and an audit of hospital guidelines. *Journal of Clinical Excellence* 2000; **2**: 161–7.
233 Hall JM, Fairney A. Audit of a dedicated osteoporosis clinic. *Journal of Clinical Effectiveness* 1998; **3**: 128–33.
234 Conning S, Fellowes D, Sheldon H. Users' views in theory and in practice. *Journal of Clinical Effectiveness* 1997; **2**: 31–4.
235 Cunningham C, Newton R. A question sheet to encourage written consultation questions. *Quality in Health Care* 2000; **9**: 42–6.
236 Grimes K. Using patients' views to improve a healthcare service. *Journal of Clinical Excellence* 2000; **2**: 99–102.
237 Kroese BS, Gillott A, Atkinson V. Consumers with intellectual disabilities as service evaluators. *Journal of Applied Research in Intellectual Disabilities* 1998; **11**: 116–28.
238 Antrobus H. Do-it-yourself pain control. *ImpAct* 1999; **1**: 6–7.
239 Hall W, Violato C, Lewkonia R, Lockyer J, Fidler H, Toews J *et al.* Assessment of physician performance in Alberta: the physician achievement review. *Canadian Medical Assocation Journal* 1999; **161**: 52–7.
240 Judd M. A pragmatic approach to user involvement in clinical audit making it happen. *Journal of Clinical Effectiveness* 1997; **2**: 35–8.
241 Bain J, Kelly H, Snadden D, Staines H. Day surgery in Scotland: patient satisfaction and outcomes. *Quality in Health Care* 1999; **8**: 86–91.
242 Poulton BC. User involvement in identifying health needs and shaping and evaluating services: is it being realised? *Journal of Advanced Nursing* 1999; **30**: 1289–96.

243 Stevenson K. Warm soft fuzzies? Is there a problem involving patients in audit? *Audit Trends* 1997; **5**: 1–3.

244 Gilbert D. Involving patients: lessons from PACE. (PACE series (Promoting Action on Clinical Effectiveness). Reasons for involving patients in care and treatment decisions). *Nursing Times* 1998; –9.

245 Cates C. Promoting interest in evidence-based practice in primary care. *ImpAct* 2000; **2**: 1–3.

246 Lindstrom K, Berg L, Rylander B, Hagman A, Olsson L, Bengtsson C. A model for quality assessment in primary healthcare using the tracer condition technique with insulin treated diabetes as one of the tracers. *Scandinavian Journal of Primary Health Care* 1997; **15**: 92–6.

247 Robinson RO, Edwards M, Madigan C, Ledgar S, Boutros A. Audit of a children's epilepsy clinic. *Developmental Medicine & Child Neurology* 2000; **42**: 387–91.

248 Jones A. Joint audit of referral letters and discharge summaries in the Hastings district. *Audit Trends* 1996; **4**: 5–10.

249 Burrow J, Rimmer JW. Accuracy of medication records for patients with learning difficulties: an interface audit between the Phoenix NHS Trust and Avon Primary Care Audit Group. *Journal of Clinical Effectiveness* 1997; **2**: 3–5.

250 Holden J. Delay pattern analysis: prospective study of alcohol problems and endocrine conditions. *Audit Trends* 1997; **5**: 121–4.

251 Robinson L, Drinkwater C. A significant case audit of a community based elderly resource team an opportunity for multidisciplinary teams to introduce clinical governance? *Journal of Clinical Governance* 2000; **8**: 89–96.

252 Westcott R, Sweeney G, Stead J. Significant event audit in practice: a preliminary study. *Family Practice* 2000; **17**: 173–9.

253 Redpath L, Stacey A, Pugh E, Holmes E. Use of the critical incident technique in primary care in the audit of deaths by suicide. *Quality in Health Care* 1997; **6**: 25–8.

254 Leape LL, Kabcenell AI, Gandhi TK, Carver P, Nolan TW, Berwick DM. Reducing adverse drug events: lessons from a breakthrough series collaborative. *Joint Commission Journal on Quality Improvement* 2000; **26**: 321–31.

255 Ash J. Multi-disciplinary audit and the mental health nurse. *Mental Health Care* 1997; **1**: 58–60.

256 Bodner C, Vale L, Ratcliffe J, Farrar S. Using economics alongside medical audit. A case study of the management of endometriosis. *Health Bulletin* 1996; **54**: 204–11.

257 Cuschieri A. Human reliability assessment in surgery – a new approach for improving surgical performance and clinical outcome. *Annals of the Royal College of Surgeons of England* 2000; **82**: 83–7.

258 Earl-Slater A, Wilcox V. Audit: an exploration of two models from outside the healthcare environment. *Journal of Evaluation in Clinical Practice* 1997; **3**: 265–74.

259 Eliasson G, Berg L, Carlsson P, Lindstrom K, Bengtsson C. Facilitating quality improvement in primary healthcare by practice visiting. *Quality in Health Care* 1998; 7: 48–54.
260 Herman A, Dreazen E, Maymon R, Tovbin Y, Bukovsky I, Weinraub Z. Implementation of nuchal translucency image-scoring method during ongoing audit. *Ultrasound in Obstetrics & Gynecology* 1999; **14**: 388–92.
261 O'Neill D, Miles A, Polychronis A. Central dimensions of clinical practice evaluation: efficiency, appropriateness and effectiveness. *Journal of Evaluation in Clinical Practice* 1996; **2**: 13–27.
262 Pitt D. Improving performance through self-assessment. *International Journal of Health Care Quality Assurance* 1999; **12**: 45–53.
263 Tourish D, Hargie O. Communication audits and the management of change: a case study from an NHS unit of management. *Health Services Management Research* 1996; **9**: 125–35.
264 Tyson SF, Turner G. The process of stroke rehabilitation: what happens and why. *Clinical Rehabilitation* 1999; **13**: 322–32.
265 Whitford DL, Scott TA. Quality improvement in the prevention of thromboembolic complications in atrial fibrillation. *Journal of Clinical Governance* 2000; **8**: 102–6.
266 Balas EA, Zong RL, Spencer DC, Jaffrey F. An expert system for performance-based direct delivery of published clinical evidence. *Journal of the American Medical Informatics Association* 1996; **3**: 56–65.
267 Cousins DD. Developing a uniform reporting system for preventable adverse drug events. *Clinical Therapeutics* 1998; **20 Suppl C**: C45–C58.
268 Wilson JD, French R, Branch T, Sutton J. Inadequate cervical cytology – the need to audit individual smear takers' inadequate rates. *Cytopathology* 1999; **10**: 107–11.
269 Sohn MJ, Byrne JV. A computerised relational database for auditing endovascular treatment of patients with intracranial aneurysms. *Neuroradiology* 2000; **42**: 762–5.
270 Kalayi C, Rimmier F, Maxwell M. Improving referral for cardiac rehabilitation – an interface audit. *Journal of Clinical Governance* 1999; **7**: 177–80.
271 Lyons C, Thomson A, Emmanuel J, Sharma R, Robertson D. Transferring cardiology out-patient follow-up from secondary to primary care. *Journal of Clinical Governance* 1999; **7**: 52–6.
272 Farrington W, Bromwich E, Cosgrove C, Walker A, Wilkins D. Improving discharge communication to general practitioners. *Audit Trends* 1998; **6**: 59–62.
273 O'Brien C, Cambouropoulos P. Combating information overload: a six-month pilot evaluation of a knowledge management system in general practice. *British Journal of General Practice* 2000; **50**: 489–90.
274 Denton AS, Bond SJ, Matthews S, Bentzen SM, Maher EJ. National audit of the management and outcome of carcinoma of the cervix treated with radiotherapy in 1993. *Clinical Oncology* 2000; **12**: 347–53.

275 Bennett J, Coles J. *Evaluating Audit: Brighton Health Care clinical audit programme: a case study*. London, CASPE, 1996.
276 Foster J, Willmot M, Coles J. *Evaluating Audit: nursing and therapy audit: an evaluation of twenty four projects and initiatives*. London, CASPE, 1996.
277 Rumsey M, Buttery Y, Bennett J, Coles J. *Wythenshawe Hospital's Clinical Audit Programme. A case study*. London, CASPE Research, 1996.
278 Rumsey M, Buttery Y, Bennett J, Coles J. *North Staffordshire's Joint Clinical Audit Programme. A case study*. London, CASPE Research, 1996.
279 Morrell C, Harvey G, Kitson A. Practitioner based quality improvement : a review of the Royal College of Nursing's dynamic standard setting system. *Quality in Health Care* 1997; **6**: 29–34.
280 Dickinson K, Edwards J. Clinical audit: failure or hidden success? *Journal of Clinical Excellence* 1999; **1**: 97–100.
281 Fraser R, Baker R. The Clinical Audit Programme in England: achievements and challenges. *Audit Trends* 1997; **5**: 131–6.
282 Johnston G, Crombie IK, Davies HTO, Alder EM, Millard A. Reviewing audit: barriers and facilitating factors for effective clinical audit. *Quality in Health Care* 2000; **9**: 23–36.
283 Newman DW, Kellett S. Clinical governance in the psychology clinic: Development of an in-house audit and evaluation system. *Journal of Clinical Governance* 2000; **8**: 21–6.
284 Redfern SJ, Norman IJ. Clinical audit, related cycles and types of healthcare quality: a preliminary model. *International Journal for Quality in Health Care* 1996; **8**: 331–40.
285 McErlain-Burns TL, Thomson R. The lack of integration of clinical audit and the maintenance of medical dominance within British hospital trusts. *Journal of Evaluation in Clinical Practice* 1999; **5**: 323–33.
286 Johanson R, Rigby C. Clinical governance in practice: achieving sustainable quality in maternity. *Journal of Clinical Excellence* 1999; **1**: 19–22.
287 Chambers R, Knight F, Campbell I. A pilot study of the introduction of audit into nursing homes. *Age and Ageing* 1996; **25**: 465–9.
288 Hearnshaw H, Reddish S, Carlyle D, Baker R, Robertson N. Introducing a quality improvement programme to primary health teams. *Quality in Health Care* 1998; **7**: 200–8.
289 Harvey G, Kitson A. Achieving improvement through quality: an evaluation of key factors in the implementation process. *Journal of Advanced Nursing* 1996; **24**: 185–95.
290 Stevenson K, Baker R, Farooqi A, Sorrie R, Khunti K. Features of primary healthcare teams associated with successful quality improvement of diabetes care. *Family Practice* 2001.
291 Carson M, Fairhead R, Rush J, Wood J. Effects and benefits of clinical audit within a multidisciplinary team. *British Journal of Therapy & Rehabilitation* 1996; **3**: 514–7.

292 Bell CM, Ma M, Campbell S, Basnett I, Pollock A, Taylor I. Methodological issues in the use of guidelines and audit to improve clinical effectiveness in breast cancer in one United Kingdom health region. *European Journal of Surgical Oncology* 2000; **26**: 130–6.

293 Berger A. Action on clinical audit: progress report. *British Medical Journal* 1998; **316**: 1893–4.

294 Stubbs K, Bhowmik P. A Quality Initiative. *Journal of Clinical Governance* 1999; 7: 62–7.

295 Fonseca S, Borgstein B, Dobson M, Hall D. The relationship between audit, research and policy: lessons from a community paediatric audiology service. *Child: Care, Health & Development* 1997; **23**: 63–76.

296 Warren B. Developing practice through clinical audit. *Journal of Clinical Effectiveness* 1998; **3**: 151–5.

297 Walshe K and Spurgeon P. *Clinical Audit Assessment Framework*. 24. Birmingham, HMSC, University of Birmingham, 1997. Handbook Series.

298 Bothner U, Georgieff M, Schwilk B. Building a large-scale perioperative anaesthesia outcome-tracking database: methodology, implementation, and experiences from one provider within the German quality project. *British Journal of Anaesthesia* 2000; **85**: 271–80.

299 Thomson R, Elcoat C, Pugh E. Clinical audit and the purchaser-provider interaction: different attitudes and expectations in the United Kingdom. *Quality in Health Care* 1996; **5**: 97–103.

300 Cheater FM, Keane M. Nurses' participation in audit: a regional study. *Quality in Health Care* 1998; **7**: 27–36.

301 Chambers R, Bowyer I, Campbell I. Investigation into the attitude of general practitioners in Staffordshire to medical audit. *Quality in Health Care* 1996; **5**: 13–9.

302 Currie IS, Paterson-Brown S. Clinical audit; who is auditing who? *Scottish Medical Journal* 1998; **43**: 185–8.

303 Millard AD, MacArthur S, McLackland D. Participation levels in local clinical audit: a pilot study comparison between healthcare professionals. *Journal of Clinical Effectiveness* 1998; **3**: 80–3.

304 Eccles M, Deverill M, McColl E, Richardson H. A national survey of audit activity across the primary secondary care interface. *Quality in Health Care* 1996; **5**: 193–200.

305 Hearnshaw H, Baker R, Cooper A. A survey of audit activity in general practice. *British Journal of General Practice* 1998; 979–81.

306 Kozlowski D. Is audit a task for nurses? *Nursing Times* 1998; **94**: 54–5.

307 Khunti K, Baker R, Rumsey M, Lakhani M. Approaches to the organization of multi-practice audits in primary healthcare in the UK. *International Journal for Quality in Health Care* 1999; **11**: 221–6.

308 Watkins CJ, King J. Understanding the barriers to medical audit: Insights from the experience of one practice. *Audit Trends* 2000; **4**: 47–52.

309 Barklie S, Stevenson K. Why do some practices fall behind schedule when undertaking a multipractice audit? Lessons for Clinical Governance. *Journal of Clinical Governance* 1999; **7**: 185.
310 Lewis C, Combes D. Is general practice audit alive and well? The view from Portsmouth. *British Journal of General Practice* 1996; **46**: 735–6.
311 Ali S. Problems doing audit for summative assessment – a general practitioner registrar's perspective. *Audit Trends* 1997; **5**: 108–10.
312 Auplish S. Using clinical audit to promote evidence-based medicine and clinical effectiveness – an overview of one health authority's experience. *Journal of Evaluation* 1997; **3**: 77–82.
313 Sealey C. Two common pitfalls in clinical audit: failing to complete the audit cycle and confusing audit with research. *British Journal of Occupational Therapy* 1999; **62**: 238–43.
314 Johnston G, Davies HTO, Crombie IK. Improving care or professional advantage? What makes clinicians do audit and how well do they fare? *Health Bulletin* 2000; **58**: 276–85.
315 Panton R, Fitzpatrick R. The involvement of pharmicists in professional and clinical audit in the UK: a review and assessment of their potential role. *Journal of Evaluation in Clinical Practice* 1996; **2**: 193–8.
316 Baxter T. Perceived barriers to promoting clinical effectiveness: a survey of clinical teams in an English health district. *Audit Trends* 1998; 8–11.
317 Greenwood JP, Lindsay SJ, Batin PD, Robinson MB. Junior doctors and clinical audit. *Journal of the Royal College of Physicians of London* 1997; **31**: 648–51.
318 Robinson S. Audit in the therapy professions: some constraints on progress. *Quality in Health Care* 1996; **5**: 206–14.
319 Johnston GN, Crombie IK, Davies HT. What stops effective clinical audit? Reports from the front line. *Scottish Medical Journal* 2000; **45**: 23–7.
320 Higginson IJ, Hearn J, Webb D. Audit in palliative care: does practice change? *European Journal of Cancer Care* 1996; **5**: 233–6.
321 McCarthy MJ, Byrne G. Surgical audit: the junior doctors' viewpoint. *Journal of the Royal College of Surgeons of Edinburgh* 1997; **42**: 317–8.
322 Robinson MB, Thompson E, Black NA. Why is evaluation of the cost effectiveness of audit so difficult? The example of thrombolysis for suspected acute myocardial infarction. *Quality in Health Care* 1998; **7**: 19–26.
323 Dolan MJ. A study of demand and need for CPD courses in clinical audit and research. *British Journal of Therapy & Rehabilitation* 1998; **5**: 511–4.
324 Miles A, Bentley P, Polychronis A, Price N, Grey J. Clinical audit in the National Health Service: fact or fiction? *Journal of Evaluation in Clinical Practice* 1996; **2**: 29–35.
325 Cranney M, Barton S, Walley T. Auditing the management of hypertension in British general practice: a critical literature review. *British Journal of General Practice* 1998; **48**: 1424–8.
326 Lough JR, Murray TS. Training for audit: lessons still to be learned. *British Journal of General Practice* 1997; **47**: 290–2.

327 Hopkins A. Clinical audit: time for a reappraisal? *Journal of the Royal College of Physicians of London* 1996; **30**: 415–25.
328 Johnstone PW, Wright J. Promoting evidence-based practice through commissioning: results of a national workshop. *Journal of Clinical Excellence* 1999; **1**: 9–12.
329 Mills K. Organisation of Health Promotion Audit in One District: Lessons from Warwickshire. *Audit Trends* 1998; **6**: 96–102.
330 Lough JR, Willmot M, Murray TS. Supporting practice-based audit: a price to be paid for collecting data. *British Journal of General Practice* 1999; **49**: 793–5.
331 Earnshaw JJ. Auditing audit: the cost of the emperor's new clothes. *Hospital Medicine* 1997; **58**: 189–92.
332 Jiwa M, Mathers N. Auditing the use of ACE inhibitors in hypertension. Reflecting the cost of clinical governance? *Journal of Clinical Governance* 2000; 27–30.
333 Robinson MB, Thompson E, Black NA. A model for estimating the cost-utility of clinical audit: the example of thrombolysis for suspected myocardial infarction. *International Journal of Technology Assessment in Health Care* 1998; **14**: 161–71.
334 Lord J, Littlejohns P. Evaluating healthcare policies: the case of clinical audit. *British Medical Journal* 1997; **315**: 668–71.
335 Millard AD. Measuring the quality of clinical audit projects. *Journal of Evaluation in Clinical Practice* 2000; **6**: 359–70.
336 Lord J, Littlejohns P. Development of an instrument to assess staff perceptions of the impact of trust-based clinical audit programmes. *Journal of Clinical Effectiveness* 1996; **1**: 83–9.
337 Balogh R, Quinn H, Simpson A, Bond S. A comparative analysis of six audit systems for mental health nursing. *International Journal for Quality in Health Care* 1998; **10**: 43–52.
338 Millard AD. Simple is best: a review of some audit quality measures. *Journal of Clinical Excellence* 1999; **1**: 23–6.
339 Semple DM, Khaled K, Maresh MJA. Monitoring quality of audit in obstetrics and gynaecology. *Quality in Health Care* 2000; **9**: 37–41.
340 Gillies A. Improving patient care in the UK: clinical audit in the Oxford Region. *International Journal for Quality in Health Care* 1996; **8**: 141–52.
341 Houghton G, O'Mahoney D, Sturman SG, Unsworth J. The clinical implementation of clinical governance: acute stroke management as an example. *Journal of Clinical Excellence* 1999; **1**: 129–32.
342 McConachie HR. Conceptual frameworks in evaluation of multidisciplinary services for children with disabilities. *Child: Care, Health & Development* 1999; **25**: 101–13.
343 Miles A, Bentley P, Price N, Polychronis A, Grey J, Asbridge J. The Total Health Care Audit System: a systematic methodology for clinical practice evaluation and development in NHS provider organizations. *Journal of Evaluation in Clinical Practice* 1996; **2**: 37–64.

344 Balas EA, Boren SA, Brown GD, Ewigman BG, Mitchell JA, Perkoff GT. Effect of physician profiling on utilization. Meta-analysis of randomized clinical trials. *Journal of General Internal Medicine* 1996; **11**: 584–90.
345 Mugford M, Banfield P, O'Hanlon M. Effects of feedback of information on clinical practice: a review. *British Medical Journal* 1991; **303**: 398–402.
346 Thomson O'Brien MA, Oxman AD, Davis DA, Haynes RB, Freemantle N, Harvey EL. Audit and feedback: effects on professional practice and healthcare outcomes. *Cochrane Database of Systematic Reviews* 2000; **Issue 2, 2000**.
347 Anderson GM, Lexchin J. Strategies for improving prescribing practice. *Canadian Medical Assocation Journal* 1996; **154**: 1013–7.
348 Aspegren K. Teaching and learning communication skills in medicine: a review with quality grading of articles. *Medical Teacher* 1999; **21**: 563–70.
349 Beilby JJ, Silagy CA. Trials of providing costing information to general practitioners: a systematic review. *Medical Journal of Australia* 1997; **167**: 89–92.
350 Bordley WC, Chelminski A, Margolis PA, Kraus R, Szilagyi PG, Vann JJ. The effect of audit and feedback on immunization delivery: a systematic review. *American Journal of Preventive Medicine* 2000; **18**: 343–50.
351 Buntinx F, Winkens R, Grol R, Knottnerus JA. Influencing diagnostic and preventive performance in ambulatory care by feedback and reminders. A review. *Family Practice* 1993; **10**: 219–28.
352 Thomson O'Brien MA, Oxman AD, Davis DA, Haynes RB, Freemantle N, Harvey EL. Audit and feedback versus alternative strategies: effects on professional practice and healthcare outcomes. *Cochrane Database of Systematic Reviews* 2000; **Issue 2, 2000**.
353 Lloyd JS, Abrahamson S. Effectiveness of continuing medical education: a review of the evidence. *Evaluation & the Health Professions* 1979; **2**: 251–80.
354 Freudenstein U, Howe A. Recommendations for future studies: a systematic review of educational interventions in primary care settings. *British Journal of General Practice* 1999; **49**: 995–1001.
355 Hanson LC, Tulsky JA, Danis M. Can clinical interventions change care at the end of life? *Annals of Internal Medicine* 1997; **126**: 381–8.
356 Thomson O'Brien MA, Oxman AD, Davis DA, Haynes RB, Freemantle N, Harvey EL. Educational outreach visits: effects on professional practice and healthcare outcomes. *Cochrane Database of Systematic Reviews* 2000; **Issue 2, 2000**.
357 Thomson O'Brien MA, Oxman AD, Haynes RB, Davis DA, Freemantle N, Harvey EL. Local opinion leaders: effects on professional practice and healthcare outcomes. *Cochrane Database of Systematic Reviews* 2000; **Issue 2, 2000**.
358 Balas EA, Austin SM, Mitchell JA, Ewigman BG, Bopp KD, Brown GD. The clinical value of computerized information services. A review of 98 randomized clinical trials. *Archives of Family Medicine* 1996; **5**: 271–8.
359 Yano EM, Fink A, Hirsch SH, Robbins AS, Rubenstein LV. Helping practices reach primary care goals. Lessons from the literature. *Archives of Internal Medicine* 1995; **155**: 1146–56.

360 Bower P. On-site mental health workers in primary care: effects on professional practice. *Cochrane Database of Systematic Reviews* 2001; **Issue 1, 2001**.
361 Shortell SM, Bennett CL, Byck GR. Assessing the impact of continuous quality improvement on clinical practice: what it will take to accelerate progress. *Milbank Quarterly* 1998; **76**: 593–624.
362 Chaix-Couturier C, Durand-Zaleski I, Jolly D, Durieux P. Effects of financial incentives on medical practice: Results from a systematic review of the literature and methodological issues. *International Journal for Quality in Health Care* 2000; **12**: 133–42.
363 Davis DA, Taylor-Vaisey A. Translating guidelines into practice. A systematic review of theoretic concepts, practical experience and research evidence in the adoption of clinical practice guidelines. *Canadian Medical Assocation Journal* 1997; **157**: 408–16.
364 Davis DA, Thomson MA, Oxman AD. Changing physician performance: a systematic review of the effect of continuing medical education strategies. *Journal of the American Medical Association* 1995; **274**: 700–5.
365 Oxman AD, Thomson MA, Davis DA, Haynes RB. No magic bullets: a systematic review of 102 trials of interventions to improve professional practice. *Canadian Medical Assocation Journal* 1995; **153**: 1423–31.
366 Smith WR. Evidence for the effectiveness of techniques to change physician behavior. *Chest* 2000; **118**: 8S–17S.
367 Thomas LH, McColl E, Cullum N, Rousseau N, Soutter J. Clinical guidelines in nursing, midwifery, and the therapies: a systematic review. *Journal of Advanced Nursing* 1999; **30**: 40–50.
368 Wensing M, Van der WT, Grol R. Implementing guidelines and innovations in general practice: which interventions are effective? *British Journal of General Practice* 1998; **48**: 991–7.
369 NHS Centre for Reviews and Dissemination. Implementing clinical guidelines: can guidelines be used to improve clinical practice? *Effective Health Care* 1994; **1**(8).
370 Mandelblatt J, Kanetsky PA. Effectiveness of interventions to enhance physician screening for breast cancer. *Journal of Family Practice* 1995; **40**: 162–71.
371 Soumerai SB, McLaughlin TJ, Avorn J. Improving drug prescribing in primary care: a critical analysis of the experimental literature. *Milbank Quarterly* 1989; **67**: 268–317.
372 Freemantle N, Harvey EL, Wolf F, Grimshaw JM, Grilli R, Bero LA. Printed educational materials: effects on professional practice and healthcare outcomes. *Cochrane Database of Systematic Reviews* 2000; **Issue 2, 2000**.
373 Gill PS, Makela M, Vermeulen KM, Freemantle N, Ryan G, Bond C *et al.* Changing doctor prescribing behaviour. *Pharmacy World & Science* 1999; **21**: 158–67.
374 Lomas J, Haynes RB. A taxonomy and critical review of tested strategies for the application of clinical practice recommendations: from 'official' to 'individual' clinical policy. *American Journal of Preventive Medicine* 1988; **2**: 77–94.

375 Worrall G, Chaulk P, Freake D. The effects of clinical practice guidelines on patient outcomes in primary care: a systematic review. *Canadian Medical Assocation Journal* 1997; **156**: 1705–12.
376 Hulscher MEJL. Interventions to implement prevention in primary care. *Cochrane Database of Systematic Reviews* 2001; **Issue 1, 2001**.
377 Kroenke K, Taylor-Vaisey A, Dietrich AJ, Oxman TE. Interventions to improve provider diagnosis and treatment of mental disorders in primary care. *Psychosomatics* 2000; **41**: 39–52.
378 Renders CM, Valk GD, Griffin S, Wagner EH, van Eijk JThM, Assendelft WJJ. Interventions to improve the management of diabetes mellitus in primary care, outpatient and community settings. *Cochrane Database of Systematic Reviews* 2001; **Issue 1, 2001**.
379 Solomon DH, Hashimoto H, Daltroy L, Liang MH. Techniques to improve physicians' use of diagnostic tests: a new conceptual framework. *Journal of the American Medical Association* 1998; **280**: 2020–7.
380 Gyorkos TW, Tannenbaum TN, Abrahamowicz M. Evaluation of the effectiveness of immunisation delivery methods. *Canadian Journal of Public Health* 1994; **85**: S14–S30.
381 Snell JL, Buck EL. Increasing cancer screening: meta analysis. *Preventive Medicine* 1996; **25**: 702–7.
382 Austin SM, Balas EA, Mitchell JA, Ewigman BG. Effect of physician reminders on preventive care: meta-analysis of randomized clinical trials. *Proceedings of the Annual Symposium on Computer Applications in Medical Care* 1994; 121–4.
383 Balas EA, Weingarten S, Garb CT, Blumenthal D, Boren SA, Brown GD. Improving preventive care by prompting physicians. *Archives of Internal Medicine* 2000; **160**: 301–8.
384 Shea S, DuMouchel W, Bahamonde L. A meta-analysis of 16 randomized controlled trials to evaluate computer-based clinical reminder systems for preventive care in the ambulatory setting. *Journal of the American Medical Informatics Association* 1996; **3**: 399–409.
385 Shiffman RN, Liaw Y, Brandt CA, Corb GJ. Computer-based guideline implementation systems: a systematic review of functionality and effectiveness. *Journal of the American Medical Informatics Association* 1999; **6**: 104–14.
386 Sullivan F, Mitchell E. Has general practitioner computing made a difference to patient care? A systematic review of published reports. *British Medical Journal* 1995; **311**: 848–52.
387 Walton RT, Harvey E, Dovey S, Freemantle N. Computerised advice on drug dosage to improve prescribing practice. *Cochrane Database of Systematic Reviews* 2001; **Issue 1, 2001**.
388 Hunt DL, Haynes RB, Hanna SE, Smith K. Effects of computer-based clinical decision support systems on physician performance and patient outcomes: a systematic review. *Journal of the American Medical Association* 1998; **280**: 1339–46.

389 Colombet I, Chatellier G, Jaulent MC, Degoulet P. Decision aids for traige of patients with chest pain: a systematic review of field evaulation studies. *Proceedings of the AMIA Annual Symposium* 1999; 721–5.
390 Davis D, O'Brien MA, Freemantle N, Wolf FM, Mazmanian P, Taylor-Vaisey A. Impact of formal continuing medical education: do conferences, workshops, rounds, and other traditional continuing education activities change physician behavior or healthcare outcomes? *Journal of the American Medical Association* 1999; **282**: 867–74.
391 Beaudry JS. The effectiveness of continuing medical education: a quantitative synthesis. *Journal of Continuing Education in the Health Professions* 1989; **9**: 285–307.
392 Bertram DA, Brooks-Bertram PA. The evaluation of continuing medical education: a literature review. *Health Education Monographs* 1977; **5**: 330–62.
393 Waddell DL. The effects of continuing education on nursing practice: a meta-analysis. *Journal of Continuing Education in Nursing* 1991; **22**: 113–18.
394 Currell R. Nursing record systems: effects on nursing practice and healthcare outcomes. *Cochrane Database of Systematic Reviews* 2001; **Issue 1, 2001**.
395 Lancaster T, Silagy C, Fowler G. Training health professionals in smoking cessation. *Cochrane Database of Systematic Reviews* 2001; **Issue 1, 2001**.
396 Gurwitz JH, Soumerai SB, Avorn J. Improving medication prescribing and utilization in the nursing home. *Journal of the American Geriatrics Society* 1990; **38**: 542–52.
397 Zwarenstein M. Interprofessional education: effects on professional practice and healthcare outcomes. *Cochrane Database of Systematic Reviews* 2001; **Issue 1, 2001**.
398 Zwarenstein M. Interventions to promote collaboration between nurses and doctors. *Cochrane Database of Systematic Reviews* 2000; **Issue 2, 2000**.
399 Giuffrida A, Pedersen L. Target payments in primary care: effects on professional practice and healthcare outcomes. *Cochrane Database of Systematic Reviews* 2001; **Issue 1, 2001**.
400 Gosden T, Forland F, Kristiansen IS, Sutton M, Leese B, Giuffrida A *et al.* Capitation, salary, fee-for-service and mixed systems of payment: effects on the behaviour of primary care physicians. *Cochrane Database of Systematic Reviews* 2001; **Issue 1, 2001**.
401 Grilli R, Freemantle N, Minozzi S, Domenighetti G, Finer D. Mass media interventions: effects on health services utilisation. *Cochrane Database of Systematic Reviews* 2000; **Issue 2, 2000**.
402 Harvey EL, Glenny A, Kirk SFL, Summerbell CD. Improving health professionals' management and the organisation of care for overweight and obese people. *Cochrane Database of Systematic Reviews* 2000; **Issue 2, 2000**.
403 Grimshaw JM. Evaluation of four quality assurance initiatives to improve outpatient referrals from general practice to hospital. *PhD Thesis* 1998.

404 Grilli R, Lomas J. Evaluating the message: the relationship between compliance rate and the subject of a practice guideline. *Medical Care* 1994; **32**: 202–13.
405 Lomas J. Words without action? The production, dissemination, and impact of consensus recommendations. *Annual Review of Public Health* 1991; **12**: 41–65.
406 Thomas L, Cullum N, McColl E, Rousseau N, Soutter J, Steen N. Guidelines in professions allied to medicine. *Cochrane Database of Systematic Reviews* 2000; **Issue 2, 2000**.

Annex 1

Key points identified in the NCCA review[2]

- It appears to be desirable that those whose work will be covered by an audit participate in selecting the subject and setting objectives for the audit, using a systematic method which focuses on important subjects for audit as perceived by the participants.
- Measures of practice can be used effectively in audit to contribute to improvements in practice when they are developed by or otherwise made acceptable to the practitioners whose performance is to be reviewed.
- Implicit measures of quality of care appear to be less reliable in audit than explicit measures.
- Measures of processes and outcomes of care or process measures alone are preferable to outcome measures alone.
- The patient medical record may be the most readily available and least costly data source for audit in many organisations; however, data from other sources may be more complete.
- A two-phased strategy of (1) using explicit criteria to measure quality of care across several cases and (2) using structured implicit criteria to review the individual cases which do not meet explicit criteria can enable practitioners to focus on potential reasons why there are cases which do not meet either explicit or implicit criteria.
- Audit leaders can motivate colleagues to improve by focusing on what can be done about obvious shortcomings in care provided to patients.
- Changes in practice may be achieved more effectively if a strategy involving several different types of action is used.

Index

adverse event, defined 69
Agency for Health Care Policy and Research (AHCPR), criteria 26
aims
  book's 1–2
  clinical audit 13–14
ankylosing spondylitis, data collection example 35
antibiotic prescribing, change implementation example 56
appendices, notes on 5–6
appraisals, health technology 71
audit *see* clinical audit

Bandolier, online resource 80
bar chart example 42
barriers
  change 49–50
  to successful audit 49–50
Beacon sites, NHS 29–30
  IT 60
  online resource 82
  quality improvement support 66
behaviour, changing 48–50
benchmarking 141–2
  criteria 28–9
  defined 69
book, how to use this 4–6
BPR *see* business process re-engineering
brainstorming, team environments 53–4
Bristol Royal Infirmary Inquiry, recommendations 2, 64–5, 119–23
  Government response 119–23
business process re-engineering (BPR), clinical audit cycle 3

CAA *see* Clinical Audit Association
Caesarian section, change implementation example 56
Cancer Services Collaborative (CSC) 37
  online resource 80
care pathways, criteria 30
CCAD *see* Central Cardiac and Audit Database
CD-ROM, book's 4, 6, 50
CEEU *see* Royal College of Physicians of England Clinical Effectiveness and Evaluation Unit
Central Cardiac and Audit Database (CCAD), data use 44
Centre for Reviews and Dissemination (CRD), online resource 78–9
CGA *see* Clinical Governance Association
CGRDU *see* Clinical Governance Research and Development Unit
CGSDU *see* Clinical Governance Support and Development Unit; Clinical Governance Support and Development Unit (Wales)
change
  barriers 49–50
  considering 145
  evaluating 60–2
  group 49
  implementing 50, 56–7, 146, 154–63
  individual 49
  monitoring 60–2
  organisational 48–9
charts, examples 42
checklists 105–13
CHI *see* Commission for Health Improvement
clinical audit
  aims 13–14
  checklists 105–13
  cycle 2–3
  defined 1, 69
  evaluating 62–3, 90–1
  online resources 73–92
  preparing 9–20
  priorities 12–14
  promoting successful 51, 150–1
  understanding 19
Clinical Audit Association (CAA), online resource 84

Clinical Effectiveness and Evaluation Unit (CEEU), online resource 89
clinical effectiveness, defined 70
clinical evidence, online resource 78
clinical governance 4
 defined 70
 system 54
Clinical Governance Association (CGA), online resource 85
Clinical Governance Research and Development Unit (CGRDU), online resource 85
Clinical Governance Support and Development Unit (CGSDU) 66
Clinical Governance Support and Development Unit (Wales) (CGSDU), online resource 85
clinical guidelines
 defined 70
 online resources 77–8
clinical performance indicators 60–2
 coronary heart disease 61–2
clinical quality improvement (CQI), clinical audit cycle 3
Clinical Resource and Audit Group (CRAG), online resource 85–6
CLIP database, online resource 80
CME *see* continuing medical education
Cochrane Library, online resource 78
College of Occupational Therapists, online resource 86–7
Commission for Health Improvement (CHI)
 clinical audit approach 115–17
 ensuring clinical audit 12
 online resource 80–1
Community Practitioners and Health Visitors Association (CPHVA), online resource 87
concurrent data collection 40–1
consumer audit, criteria 27–8
continuing medical education (CME) 161
coronary heart disease, clinical performance indicators 61–2
CPHVA *see* Community Practitioners and Health Visitors Association
CQI *see* clinical quality improvement
CRAG *see* Clinical Resource and Audit Group
CRD *see* Centre for Reviews and Dissemination
criteria
 benchmarking 28–9
 care pathways 30
 defining 22–3, 70
 developing 23–4, 24–6, 139–42
 guidelines 24
 implicit 24
 key points 21, 102
 outcome 23, 27–8
 performance levels 28
 population definition 34
 prescriptions 25
 process 23
 professional consensus 26–7
 RAND/UCLA appropriateness method 26
 review criteria, desirable characteristics 131–2
 selecting 21–32
 structure 22
 user involvement 27–8
critical incident technique, criteria 27–8
critically appraised topics, online resources 78–9
CRU *see* Royal College of Psychiatrists Research Unit
CSC *see* Cancer Services Collaborative

data
 abstraction tools 40
 analysis 41–2, 144–5
 collection 34–6, 40–1, 144–5, 148
 effective use promotion 44
 electronic capture 43
 handling 38–45
 management, staff role 16
 sources 38–9, 143–4
Data Protection Act 43–5
discussion groups, online resource 84

EFQM *see* European Foundation for Quality Management
electronic data capture 43
encouraging staff 17–19
environments
 creating 1–7
 establishing the right 52–4
 individual 52–3
 organisational 52, 54
 team 52, 53–4
Essence of Care. Patient-Focused Benchmarking for Health Care Practitioners 29
European Foundation for Quality Management (EFQM) 64
evaluating
 change 60–2
 clinical audit 62–3, 90–1
 methods 154
evidence-based practice, defined 70
evidence, review *see* review of evidence
external relationships 54–6

facilitation
  defined 71
  staff role 16
feedback 157–60
flowcharts 17–19
focus groups, criteria 27–8
force-field analysis, team environments 53–4
frameworks, using existing 63–4
Fundamentals of Care Project 29
funding 14–15
further reading 97–100

gateways, online resource 91–2
General Medical Council (GMC) 2
  data protection 44–5
glossary 69–72
GMC *see* General Medical Council
Good Practice in Clinical Audit 5
group change 49
guidelines
  clinical 70, 77–8
  criteria 24
  NGC 77
  SIGN 24, 77–8

health care organisations 55–6
Health Evidence Bulletins Wales, online resource 79
health technology appraisals, defined 71
hypertension, sample sizes example 36–7

ideas collection, team environments 53–4
IHI *see* Institute for Healthcare Improvement
IM&T *see* Information Management and Technology
ImpAct, online resource 81
implicit criteria 24
improvements
  key notes 47, 59, 104
  key points 47, 59, 103–4
  maintaining 62–6
  making 47–58
  reinforcing 62–6
  sustaining 59–67
Improving Health in Wales 55
inclusion criteria, population definition 34
individual change 49
individual environments 52–3
information
  online resources 73–92
  sources of user 11
information/knowledge support, staff role 16

Information Management and Technology (IM&T)
  impact 148–9
  using 60
Inquiry, Bristol Royal Infirmary *see* Bristol Royal Infirmary Inquiry
Institute for Healthcare Improvement (IHI), online resource 81–2
interval sampling 37
IT *see* Information Management and Technology

Joint Royal Colleges Ambulance Liaison Committee (JRCALC), online resource 87

key notes 5, 101–4
  improvements 47, 59, 104
  performance levels 33, 102–3
key points 5, 101–4
  criteria 21, 102
  improvements 47, 59, 103–4
  NCCA 191
  performance levels 33, 102–3
  preparing for audit 9, 101
knowledge management 65–6

leadership 64
learning organisation 65
Learning Zone, online resource 83
level of performance 71
Library and Information Service, online resource 86
lumbar spine radiography, setting time periods 35

management, project *see* project management
Maternity Care Data Project, data use 44
methods
  evaluating 154
  used in audit 136–49
  using the 1–7
MIQUEST
  data source 38
  data use 44

National Centre for Clinical Audit (NCCA)
  key points 190
  review 134–6, 190
National Centre for Health Outcomes Development (NHCOD), online resource 79–80
National Clinical Audit Support Programme (NCASP), data use 44
National Co-ordinating Centre for NHS Service Delivery and Organisation (NCCSDO)
  change management 48
  online resource 82

National electronic Library for Health (NeLH), online resource 77, 91–2
National Guideline Clearing House (NGC), online resource 77
National Institute for Clinical Excellence (NICE)
  online resource 77
  projects sponsored by 93–5
national involvement 12
National Patient Safety Agency, online resource 83
National Primary Care Development Team (NPDT), online resource 83
National Sentinel Audits (NSA), lessons learnt from 125–30
National Service Frameworks (NSF) 55–6
  defined 71
  online resource 79
NCASP *see* National Clinical Audit Support Programme
NCCA *see* National Centre for Clinical Audit
NCCSDO *see* National Co-ordinating Centre for NHS Service Delivery and Organisation
NCHOD *see* National Centre for Health Outcomes Development
NeLH *see* National electronic Library for Health
NGC *see* National Guideline Clearing House
NHS Beacon sites *see* Beacon sites, NHS
NHS Clinical Governance Support Team, online resource 86
NHS Plan 2
  user involvement 54–5
NICE *see* National Institute for Clinical Excellence
NMAP *see* Nursing, Midwifery and Allied Health Professionals Gateway
NPDT *see* National Primary Care Development Team
NSA *see* National Sentinel Audits
NSF *see* National Service Frameworks
Nursing, Midwifery and Allied Health Professionals Gateway (NMAP), online resource 91

OHNiP *see* Our Healthier Nation in Practice database
OMNI *see* Organising Medical Networked Information
online resources 73–92
  awareness development 74
  critical appraisal 75
  information types 74–5
organisation of audit, review of evidence 149–54
organisational change 48–9
organisational culture
  changing 64–5
  learning organisation 65
organisational development, appropriate 63
organisational environments 52, 54
Organising Medical Networked Information (OMNI), online resource 91
otitis media, change implementation example 56
Our Healthier Nation in Practice (OHNiP) database, online resource 83
outcomes
  criteria 23, 27–8
  defined 71
  evidence review 142–3
  NHCOD 79–80

PACT *see* Prescription Analysis and Cost
pain control, change implementation example 56
patient administration systems (PAS), data source 38
Patient Advocacy and Liaison Service 11, 54–5
Patient Forum 11, 54–5
Patient Support Managers 55
Performance Analysis Toolkit, data use 44
performance levels
  clinical performance indicators 60–2
  criteria 28
  key notes 33, 102–3
  key points 33, 102–3
  measuring 33–46
poor practice 12
population definition, criteria 34
preparing for audit 9–20
  elements 10
  key points 9, 101
Prescription Analysis and Cost (PACT), data source 38
prescriptions
  criteria 25
  repeat 17–19
Primary Care Information Services (PRIMIS), data use 44
priorities, clinical audit 12–14
process criteria 23
project management
  clinical audit preparation 10
  staff role 17
project methodology, clinical audit preparation 10
public, users and the 54–5

qualitative analysis 43
quality
  assurance 14
  evaluating clinical audit 62–3
  improvement 65–6

RAND/UCLA appropriateness method, criteria 26
rapid-cycle sampling 37
RCGP *see* Royal College of General Practitioners
RCN *see* Royal College of Nursing
RCOA *see* Royal College of Anaesthetists
RCOG *see* Royal College of Obstetricians and Gynaecologists
references, review of evidence 165–90
repeat prescriptions 17–19
research, defined 71
resources
  map 76
  online 73–92
retrospective data collection 40–1
review criteria, desirable characteristics 131–2
review of evidence 131–90
  change, considering 145
  change, implementing 146, 154–63
  conclusions 163–5
  criteria development 139–42
  data analysis 144–5
  data collection 144–5, 148
  data sources 143–4
  discussion 163–5
  methods used in audit 136–49
  NCCA review 132–6, 190
  organisation of audit 149–54
  outcomes 142–3
  references 165–90
  user involvement 147–8
risk adjustment, outcome criteria 23
Royal College of Anaesthetists (RCOA), online resource 87
Royal College of General Practitioners (RCGP), online resource 88
Royal College of Nursing (RCN), online resource 88
Royal College of Obstetricians and Gynaecologists (RCOG), online resource 88
Royal College of Pathologists, online resource 89
Royal College of Physicians of England Clinical Effectiveness and Evaluation Unit (CEEU), online resource 89
Royal College of Psychiatrists, priorities 13
Royal College of Psychiatrists Research Unit (CRU), online resource 89
Royal College of Radiologists, online resource 90
Royal Pharmaceutical Society (RPSGB), online resource 90

sampling
  interval 37
  rapid-cycle 37
  sample sizes 36–7
  two-stage 37
  users 36
Scottish Intercollegiate Guidelines Network (SIGN)
  guidelines 24
  online resource 77–8
Service Delivery Practice Database, online resource 84
SIGN *see* Scottish Intercollegiate Guidelines Network
skills
  developing 15, 17–19
  identifying 15
social care organisations 55–6
staff
  encouraging 17–19
  roles 16–17
  supporting 17–19
standards
  defining 22, 71
  online resources 79–80
statements, population definition 34
statistical control chart example 42
stroke, change implementation example 57
structure criteria 22
structure, need for 14
supporting staff 17–19
systematic review
  defined 72
  online resources 78–9
systems, user involvement 11

teams
  audit project 16
  clinical audit 12–14
  environments 52, 53–4
time, making 15
time periods, setting 35
total quality management (TQM), clinical audit cycle 3
training, staff role 17
two-stage sampling 37

UK Central Council for Nursing, Midwifery and Health Visiting 2
understanding clinical audit 19
urinary incontinence, data source example 39
user information, sources 11
user involvement
  criteria 27–8
  NHS Plan 54–5
  review of evidence 147–8
  systems 11
users
  defined 72
  identifying 34–6
  and the public 54–5
  sampling 36

WISDOM, online resource 86
world-wide web *see* online resources